HELLO & WELCOME TO THE BODY PLAN PLUS

The Dieting and Exercise World has become a crazy place and the fundamental message has gotten lost - Or should I dare to say pushed aside by the dieting industry?

Dieting & Exercise is about basic math and common sense!

Calories (Energy) you consume should be equal to the Calories (Energy) you burn!

And if you can work that out then you can lose weight effortlessly - **And** without noticing it! (We will explain why on the next few pages)

We should all be able to work it very easily, because all the information we need for this **Very Basic** calculation is all around us...! You can't get through the day without hearing or reading the word Calories!

It's on every Packet, Bag, Menu, Bottle, Can or Tin! - **You can't go wrong!** And if you don't have any of these items to hand - Simply _Google it_ and you get the answer in less than a few seconds.

When you track your Calories (in) against your Calories (out), you can actually say "I lost weight today"

To make it all even easier than it already is: This Body Plan Food Journal - does the work for you!

The Body Plan Plus is a clever Food Journal that keeps you organised and on track.

Using the methods set out in this Journal, you can decide on how much weight you want to lose and how fast you want to get there...

It's easy, fun and rewarding - And the best thing is, you don't have to change the foods you eat! (_well not until you are ready_) Simply get a little more organised - and take control!

If you have any questions please don't hesitate to get in touch via the website.

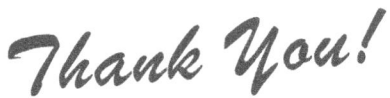

CALORIES, COUNTING OR CONTROL?

By definition: Calorie counting or Calorie control in "Dieting Terms" means counting the number of calories to be consumed. These are to be "Lower" than what your body needs to fuel itself for the day! Thus calling on your fat (Energy stores) to get you through the day. All diets work on this principle, assuming the food or diet plan structured for you is going to be lower in calories than what your body needs to fuel itself for the day.

So at the end of the day, it does not matter what diet plan or club you have joined - You are calorie counting or controlling your calories!

But why guess it?   Being on a diet plan that doesn't count calories, is like trying to run your car without a fuel gauge. All said and done, for some reason the big clubs don't want you to count your calories!

Counting your calories will give you a lot better chance of getting it right and not feeling starved, or deprived of something you like.   With technology in our hands, it's never been easier to get the calorie content of any food.
Google: "Calories in an apple" and you get the results in less than a second and you don't even need to open a web page. Record the information in your diary and you have a constant record - It's so simple!

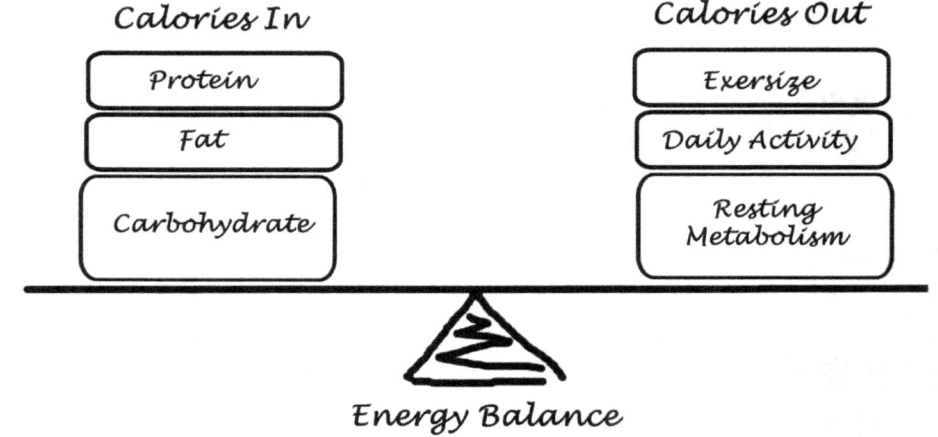

Calories In
- Protein
- Fat
- Carbohydrate

Calories Out
- Exersize
- Daily Activity
- Resting Metabolism

Energy Balance

Welcome to: The 90 Day Food & Exercise Journal - Read Me First

The Body Plan Plus 90 Day Food & Exercise Journal is divided into four sections. The first section is my "waffle" explaining various aspects of this plan, the workings and how to's. The second section is your food plan featuring your Calorie Libraries, Set Menus, Meal Planner and Food Journal Pages.

The third section of your 90 Day Journal is your exercise system starting on page 124. It's not just a "perform" these exercises kind of thing! It's a formula designed for your body type and will show you how to increase your fitness, stamina, flexibility and weight loss quickly without feeling the strain.

The fourth section is collection of Reference pages - Browse through reference when needed.

Additional Video Content

If you see a video icon at the top of any page, you can watch additional content.
Go to our Website or Facebook page, select videos and find the corresponding page number.

   www.facebook.com/the90daybodyplanplus
www.instagram.com/thebodyplanplus

Find, Like & Share! Thank You…

Now you own the Journal you are a client. So you should take advantage of client information and more. You will find the client section on our website.

Your Feedback

I would be very grateful if you could give us your feedback on your success and comment on your 90 Day Food Journal. I am keen to know how this Journal is working for you and if you could offer any suggestions and or improvements to the layout or workings. If I can gather all this feedback - maybe, together we can produce something even better? Thank You!

The Body Plan Plus TM

Front Cover/Images: Shutterstock / Wink Images
Authors: Jonathan Bowers & Angela Bowers
ISBN: See Back Cover
Printed by: Amazon

Section 1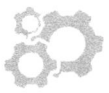

Section 2

Section 3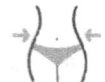

Section 4

Calorie counting and control is the key to your success. Calorie control isn't "Someone's idea of a dieting plan", it's science and just plain common sense! That is, if you understand calories in versus calories out!
I guess you already know because you're smart enough to have purchased this Journal, but just for fun, let's go over it one more time on the next page.

No matter what your goal is, to lose weight, gain weight or stay the same, calories are the most important part of your diet plan. It does not matter if your calories come from a bagel, banana or a biscuit. Calories are the key role to whether you lose, gain or maintain!

No matter what your goal is, to lose weight, gain weight or stay the same, calories are the most important part of your diet plan.
It does not matter if your calories come from a bagel, banana or a biscuit.
Calories are the key role to whether you lose, gain or maintain!

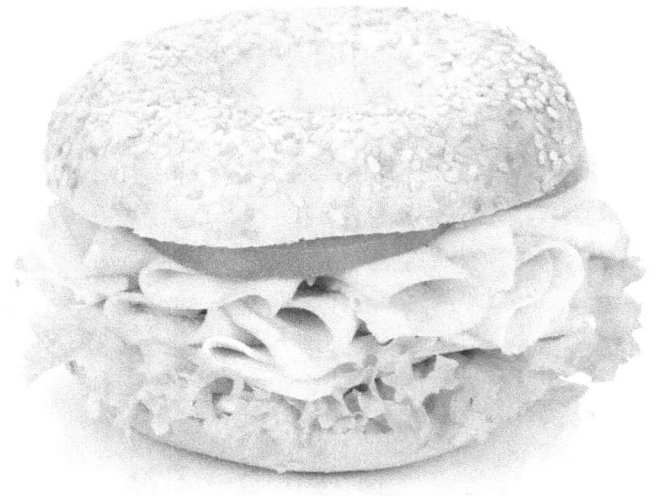

CALORIES IN AND CALORIES OUT

Calories In: With the exception of water, everything you eat or drink contains calories. Add these together and they make up your daily calorie intake. Because these calories are being consumed into your body, we refer to this as "Calories in".

Calories Out: Everything we do burns calories, and surprisingly we burn most of our calories for just being alive. Breathing, pumping blood around our bodies, digesting food, regulating our body temperature and even watching TV. This makes up for two-thirds of the calories we burn each day. This is called your Basal Metabolic Rate. (BMR)

Your BMR is the amount of calories you burn "At Rest" or doing nothing. It's a very important number and sets a bench mark for our dieting goals.

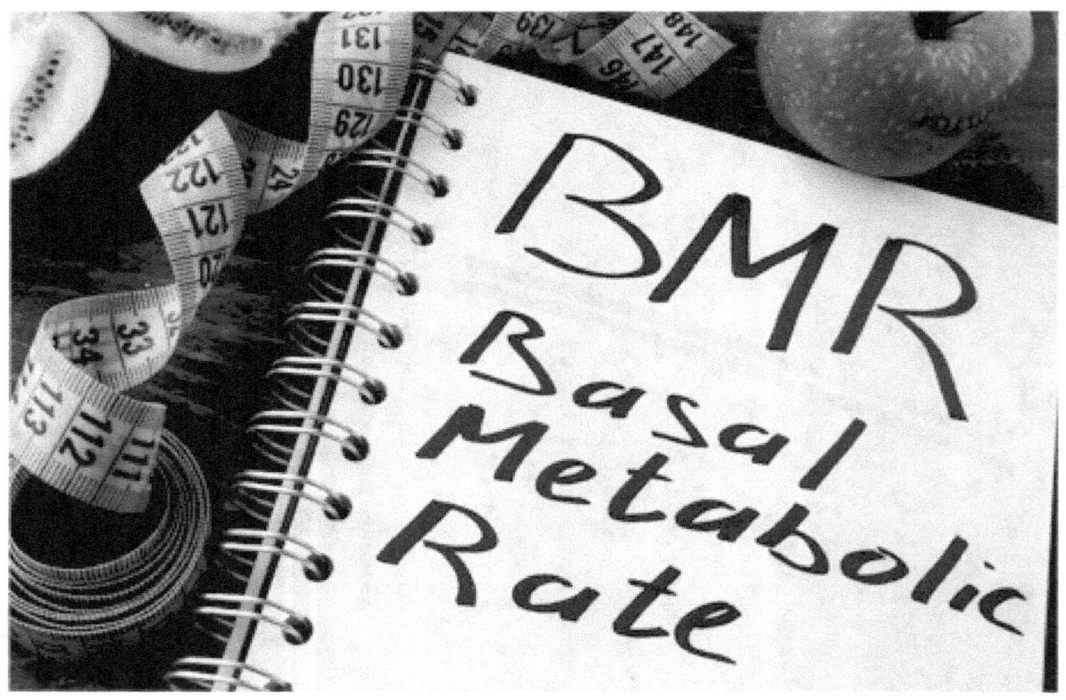

MAINTAIN, GAIN OR LOSE

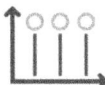

▷ Maintenance

If we get the balance right, "Calories in" matches or equals "Calories out" you will not gain or lose weight. Or put it another way, if you consume 2500 calories and burnt off 2500 calories in a single day, your body stays the same.

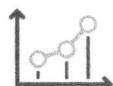

▷ Gain

Sometimes people wish to gain weight, and to do this you would consume more calories than you burn off in a single day. Or put it another way, if you consume 3000 calories and burnt off 2000 calories in a single day, your surplus would be 1000 calories. Your body has no immediate use for these extra 1000 calories, so there is only one thing it can do: store them into your body as extra fat or extra muscle.

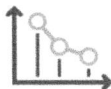

▷ Lose

This is the important part if you want to lose weight! If you want to lose weight, then your "Calories in" should be less then your "Calories out".   Or put it another way, if you consume 2000 calories, and burn off 3000 you will lose weight. You put your body into a "Calorie Deficit". In this case, 1000 calories. These extra1000 calories needed to fuel you body have to come from somewhere. So your body gets them from your fat and muscle stores from around your body. **So in a nutshell you lose weight.**

YOUR DAILY CALORIE ALLOWANCE ▶

Consuming Calories is the same for us all. Calories (Energy in) is equal, regardless of our current weight, body structure or muscle mass.

300 Calories going into someone weighing 11 stone is equal to 300 Calories going into someone who weighs 18 Stone.

But burning Calories is different! And this is why "Conventional diet plans don't work for everyone"

Our current body size, weight and muscle mass dictates how many Calories we need to fuel our body and how many Calories we burn.

The body burns Calories (Energy out) in three different forms.

1. Calories we burn for just being alive (This is our metabolic rate)
2. Calories we burn for performing day to day activities - (Walking etc)
3. Calories we burn, by forcing our muscles to work harder then normal (Exercising)

And the rate at which we burn the above **"Three"** is different for everyone!

Surprisingly we burn most of our Calories (**No.1**) for just being alive. This is called your Basal Metabolic Rate.

*Basal Metabolic Rate is the amount of energy expressed in calories that a person needs to keep the body functioning at rest. Some of those processes are breathing, blood circulation, controlling body temperature, cell growth, brain and nerve function, and contraction of muscles. Basal metabolic rate (**BMR**) affects the rate that a person burns calories and ultimately whether you maintain, gain, or lose weight. Your Basal Metabolic Rate accounts for about 60 to 75% of the calories you burn every day.*
The Harris Benedict Equation 1919 (Revised in 1984)

WE ARE ALL DIFFERENT!

So we need to work out the how many Calories - **YOUR BODY** - needs to fuel itself for the day in ratio to your current body size/weight and daily activities. As you can see from the example below, this figure can vary considerably.

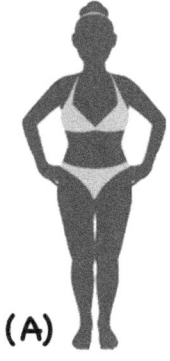

Weight: 11 Stone
Metabolic Rate - BMR   =   1400   Calories
Activity - Average   =   500   Calories
Daily Calorie Goals
Maintenance Calories   =   1900   Calories
Lose Weight Steady Pace   =   1650   Calories
Lose Weight Quick Pace   =   1400   Calories

(A)

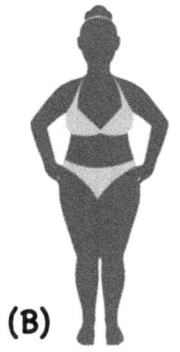

Weight: 14.6 Stone
Metabolic Rate - BMR   =   1650   Calories
Activity - Average   =   500   Calories
Daily Calorie Goals
Maintenance Calories   =   2150   Calories
Lose Weight Steady Pace   =   1900   Calories
Lose Weight Quick Pace   =   1650   Calories

(B)

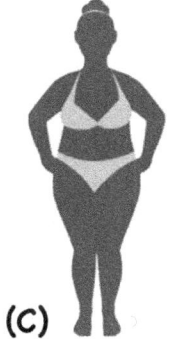

Weight: 18.5 Stone
Metabolic Rate - BMR   =   2040   Calories
Activity - Average   =   500   Calories
Daily Calorie Goals
Maintenance Calories   =   2540   Calories
Lose Weight Steady Pace   =   2290   Calories
Lose Weight Quick Pace   =   2040   Calories

(C)

As you can see we are all different and require different amounts of Calories to fuel our bodies for the day.

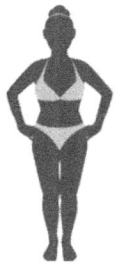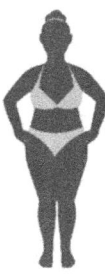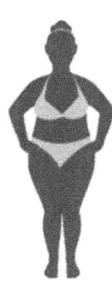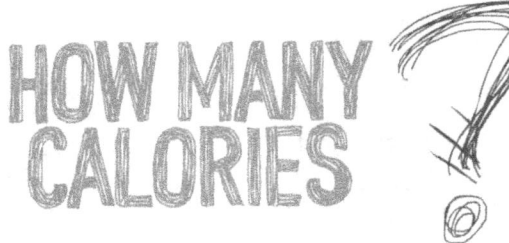

Once you know your Daily Calorie Maintenance, losing weight becomes a lot easier than simply going on a "blind, guess your calories" diet.

You now know if you consume more Calories than your **Maintenance figure** you will put weight on! This information alone will guide you to success, and you will become more aware and a lot more conscious of your Calorie intake.

You can plan your foods better, make better decisions and take complete control over your eating.

You can also, and it is advised, to play around with how many Calories you want to reduce in order to lose weight.

Some days you can reduce your calories by 500 - And this will result in a weekly loss of 1lb or more. And some days you can reduce it by 250 - or if you want a dieting break simply consume your **Maintenance figure**.

When you track, record and count your Calories, you really can say:

"I lost Weight today"

To get your Calorie Goal - Go to our website: www.thebodyplanplus.com

Scroll down to the bottom of the page, see "Clients Area" and select **BMR** Calculator. Follow the simple instructions given and enter the information required:

▷ Gender
▷ Weight
▷ Height

Activity Levels

▷ Light
▷ Moderate
▷ High

Be honest as this may effect your results. Saying you are more active than you are will result in more calories being added to your total.

You will be given two figures: Your **BMR** and Your **Daily Calorie Requirement** Level.

Your **Daily Calorie** Maintenance/*Requirement* Level here:

Your Daily **Calorie Goal** for Slow & Steady Weight Loss:

▷ To lose weight slow & steady - Reduce your Maintenance/*Requirement* level by **250** Calories

---

Your Daily **Calorie Goal** for Faster Weight Loss:

▷ To lose weight at a faster pace - Reduce your Maintenance/*Requirement* level by **500** Calories

---

▷ If you want a break from your diet programme then set your **Calorie Goal** to your Maintenance/*Requirement* Level.... Remember, if you **go over this figure** , you could be gaining weight if your activity is low!

THE 3 GOLDEN <u>FOOD</u> RULES - DO NOT! - WHY? & DO!

Food - Rule No.1

▷ **Do Not!**

Rush out and fill the shopping trolly up of the world's lowest calorie food items.

▷ **Why?**

This is what most dieters do, and it's not sustainable. You have to take it easy and swap some food items as and when the time is ready for you to do so.

▷ **Do!**

Buy what you are used to, what fits in with your family and your budget! Remember your goal is to lose body fat/weight - You are not training for a marathon!

Food - Rule No.2

▷ **Do Not!**

Set your Calorie Goal to low!

▷ **Why?**

Setting your Calorie Goal to low is not a long term solution. Your Body will notice a large reduction and it will not thank you! It will send signals to your brain asking for more!

▷ **Do!**

Play around with your Calorie Goal. Some days give yourself more and some days less. When you know your "**Daily Calorie Maintenance**" you can "Match it" go a few hundred Calories below it. We have to train your Brain to think you're not starving!

Food - Rule No.3

▷ **Do Not!**

Guess anything that passes your lips!

▷ **Why?**

The smallest of items add up… And this is where it can all go wrong big time.
A single Jelly Baby Sweet contains 22 Calories - Eating just five without thinking about is easy, but works out to be (*110 Calories*) - Going over your daily allowance by only 130 Calories can result in a yearly weight gain of 14 lbs / 1Stone!

▷ **Do!**

Track it regardless of how small or insignificant if sounds. Don't go with-out, simply track it and record it in your Journal Page. - AND YES! Even those five Jelly Babies!

Exercise - Rule No.1

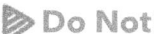 **Do Not!**

Select an Exercise starting point other than Level one! Selecting a level based on what you think is ok for you is: (Your Minds Eye Starting Point)

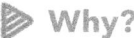 **Why?**

Regardless of what you think your current fitness level is, you should select level one. You may think after your first workout - "Well that was just so easy!" It may have been, but thats not the point - The point is you did it! Better yet, you will do it again tomorrow. It will only be a matter of days before you reach your True Body Starting Point.

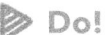 **Do!**

Move through the levels as instructed in the Exercise Programme - 3 IN A ROW!
It takes around 30 - 40 days for your Brain to associate something as "Routine in your life". Once you reach this point you have cracked it! Exercise will be built into your life! During these 30 - 40 days, the low level exercises will have kept you on the right path - Ensuring you don't hit exhaustion levels that trigger the deadly give up points!

Exercise - Rule No.2

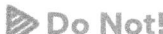 **Do Not!**

Select Exercises that are not suitable for your body type and current level of fitness.

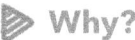 **Why?**

Selecting the wrong Exercises will simply result in you not being able to hit your Exercise time goals. This will frustrate you greatly and make you feel miserable!

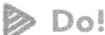 **Do!**

Try each Exercise first and see how you feel. Don't make a workout out of it, simply try them all for a few moments and be honest with how you feel. Select the Exercises that make you feel comfortable, but at the same time - Just a little challenged!

Once you have selected your Exercises, stick with them for the duration of the programme. Don't change them, until you have completed Level 16. Then repeat the process again, but this time select higher level and more intense Exercises.
If you want to know why, watch the video.   (*Clients Area / Additional Videos*)

YOUR FOOD JOURNAL PAGES

All of your food related pages are to be found in the next section of your Journal.

These pages are designed to work with each other and full details on how to use these them are about to be explained.

Your diary is organised around five main pages.

▷ *Shopping List*
▷ *Calorie Library*
▷ *Set Menus*
▷ *Meal Planner*

▷ The fifth page being your food diary page.

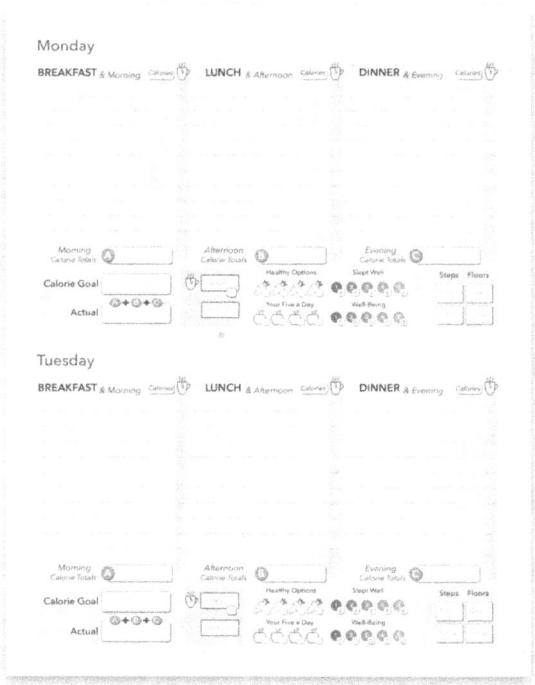

You will soon get into the flow of using these pages everyday and this will keep you organised and in control.

Shopping List

The weekly shopping list is very important and will become your guide in purchasing your food for those weeks.   Don't worry, you will not be making too many changes to begin with but simply becoming slightly more organised. After all, this is not a recipe book, we are talking about honest eating. Handy Hint - Use a pencil, because your shopping list will change.

Pages 38 to 41

Calorie Library

Don't let your calorie library confuse you. You do not need to know the calorie content for every food or each food in that group, that would by far to much for anyone. You only need to know the calorie content of the foods you eat. This is easier than ever to find out the calories and values in your food, Google will save us!

Pages 42 to 49

Set Menus

Fuss free, efficient and super simple. Set menus are really going to make your life diet friendly. Working alongside the shopping list and meal planner pages, organising your own set menus is going to make recording your food and calorie values easier than it has ever been!

Pages 50 to 55

Meal Planner

Plan your meals that you like, know and that are personal to your lifestyle. Meal planning is one of the key elements to successful dieting. If you can crack this, you are half way there. Take some time to build your meal planner and you will instantly feel organised and motivated.

Pages 56 to 69

YOUR CALORIE LIBRARY ▶

Your Calorie Library is one of the key parts to this diary and function. It's going to be a collection of the foods you eat and their calorie value. It may sound a "Hard task" to write down foods and calorie values, but trust me, it isn't. If you had to write down everything available in the supermarket, then that would be a challenge!

This is no challenge, because you only have to write down the foods that you eat. - Honest Eating.

There are four blank calorie pages, one for: Breakfast, Lunch, Dinner, Snacks & Beverages

You will find four pre-filled calorie library pages to get you started. The items featured on these pages are some of the most common used items found in the average shopping trolly.

Your blank calorie library pages will take you an hour or two to fill in, but trust me, it is well worth the effort and will make filling in your diary page really easy - And Fast!

Constantly update your calorie library every time you have something new.
Some items vary in weight, so break them down into single calorie units.
Other items, like bread slices for example are pretty standard, so simply write them down as whole values. Example given on the next page.

When you build your calorie library, use measuring spoons and measuring jug and scales. Then once you have the calculation written down in front of you.
It's so easy to refer to it.

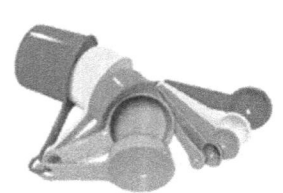 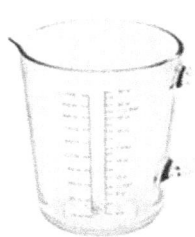 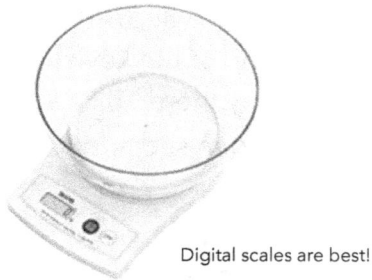

Digital scales are best!

Why everything is "Per 100 grams" or a portion size is a complete mystery to me.
It's far easier to make any calculation correctly when you simply have to "Multiply" it.
So I recommend you build your calorie library breaking down any items that
vary in weight into a single calorie unit.

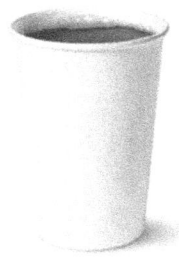

Example:
Calories in an apple per gram = 0.52 calories
Your apple slices weigh 84 grams
   84 grams x **0.52** = **43.68** Calories (Round it up to make life easy)
= **44** Calories

When you have built your own calorie library
with the foods you eat, it's so easy to refer to.
Using the Calorie Library you have created -
You would now know - for example:

Food item	Calories Per Gram
My Favourite Bread	?
My Favourite Cheese	?
My Favourite Pasta Sauce	?
My Favourite Ham Slices	?

Remember to create your Beverages library.
The calorie values for your favourite coffee
shop beverages can be found on their websites.

Remember to include all beverages, hot and cold.
And don't forget your glass of Wine!

Where possible, when preparing your meals, use your measuring cups & spoons as you
did when you created your library. This ensures your calorie value is near as spot on as
you can get it.

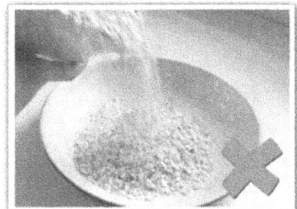 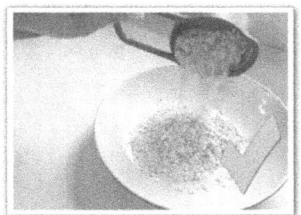 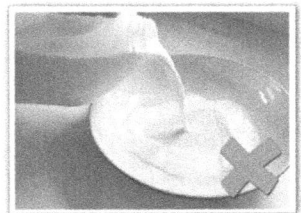 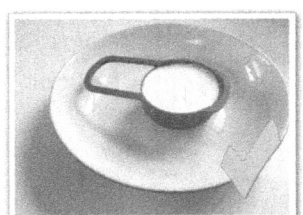

SETS MENUS

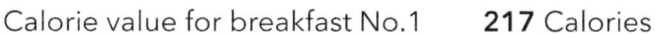 **What is a Set Menu?**

A Set menu is a collection of foods from your calorie library all bundled together for one setting.

Breakfast example:

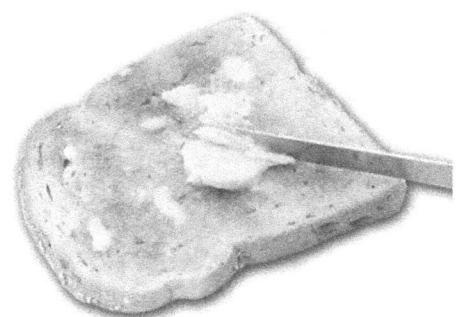

1 x Boiled egg	**78** Calories
1 x Slice of wholemeal bread	**51** Calories
1 x 5g (spoon of butter)	**37** Calories
1 x Bowl of porridge	**35** Calories
1 x Spoon of sugar	**16** Calories
Calorie value for breakfast No.1	**217** Calories

 Why have set menus?

Having a set menu will allow you to quickly calculate a pre-planned day's worth of calories. Some days you may want, or need, more calories and other days less. With your set menus, it is very easy to do this.

*For Breakfast I will have set menu No.1   Calorie Value **217***
*For Lunch I will have set menu   No.2   Calorie Value **401***
*For Dinner I will have set menu   No.3   Calorie Value **665***

Name	My Lovely Breakfast	Calories
1 x Boiled egg		78
1 x Slice/wholemeal bread		51
1 x 5g (spoon of butter)		37
1 x Bowl of porridge		35
1 x Spoon of sugar		16
Menu No. **1**	*Calorie Total*	**217**

You don't have to use your set menus all the time. They are there to make your life easy, simply for those days when you are just to busy to think about meals, and calorie calculation is far from your mind. Sometimes your set menus will simply take away the hassle of it.

I suggest you build your menus in calorie value order, from the lowest to the highest, ranging between 200 calories to700 plus calories. Having your meals vary in such calorie values will allow you to plan your days more easily. If you have a low calorie morning and afternoon, you can select a larger value evening meal.

Give your meal a name and total calorie value. When recording to your diary page, simply transfer the name and the calorie value into your calorie column.

* Your Set Menu Page   * Your Food Diary Page

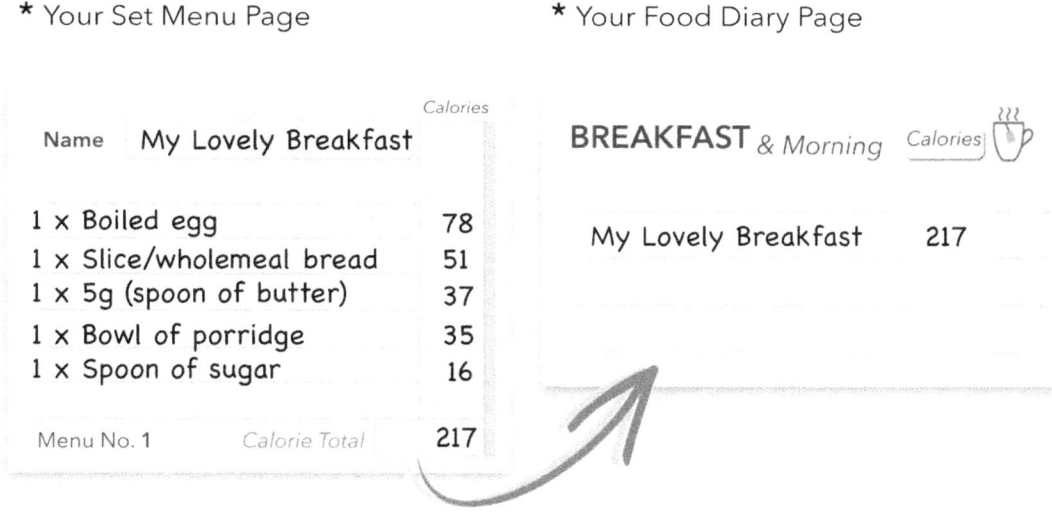

	Calories
Name My Lovely Breakfast	
1 x Boiled egg	78
1 x Slice/wholemeal bread	51
1 x 5g (spoon of butter)	37
1 x Bowl of porridge	35
1 x Spoon of sugar	16
Menu No. 1 Calorie Total	217

BREAKFAST & Morning   Calories

My Lovely Breakfast   217

There are 36 set menus in total, 12 each for Breakfast, Lunch and Dinner.
If you want to build more, you can always use your notes pages.

MEAL PLANNING

These dedicated pages are here to enable you to be more organised, which in turn will aid you in losing weight. Giving you a clear idea of what is in your food cupboard, and which day suits you best to be eating certain meals, really will benefit you.

When doing the shopping you have the necessary ingredients already outlined that you will require, whether you cook for yourself or a family. I dare say that there is even a money saving element to this in that you will no longer require to purchase those items that are not really needed. Those items like "Buy one get a third free" and in all honesty, you had no intention of buying prior to entering the store!

When you are ready to create your meal planner, using meals from your set menus or simply choosing something that is quick, simple and fits in and around your day. Here you can build your index days ahead.

QUICK VIEW MEAL PLANNER

Monday	Breakfast	Lunch	Dinner
Tuesday	Breakfast	Lunch	Dinner
Wednesday	Breakfast	Lunch	Dinner
Thursday	Breakfast	Lunch	Dinner
Friday	Breakfast	Lunch	Dinner
Saturday	Breakfast	Lunch	Dinner
Sunday	Breakfast	Lunch	Dinner

QUICK VIEW MEAL PLANNER

Monday	Breakfast	Lunch	Dinner
Tuesday	Breakfast	Lunch	Dinner
Wednesday	Breakfast	Lunch	Dinner
Thursday	Breakfast	Lunch	Dinner
Friday	Breakfast	Lunch	Dinner
Saturday	Breakfast	Lunch	Dinner
Sunday	Breakfast	Lunch	Dinner

Your meal planner will work super well for you if you have forthcoming engagements or meals out for example. You can plan the morning and lunch time meals to be lower in calories, allowing you more for the evening.
It's simple little tips and tricks like this that will keep your organised and staying within your daily calorie allowance.

You don't want to be to super enthusiastic at the start, there is no need to fill up all your Meal Planner pages with super low, celery crunching meals from the off!

This will not work, and is not honest eating. Your body requires calories so don't set your body against you.

Only fill your planner up a few days at a time or one week maximum and slowly make the changes when you are ready too.

This allows you to make changes easily, simply it gives you time to get into the swing of things!

Take some time and think carefully about your meal planning!

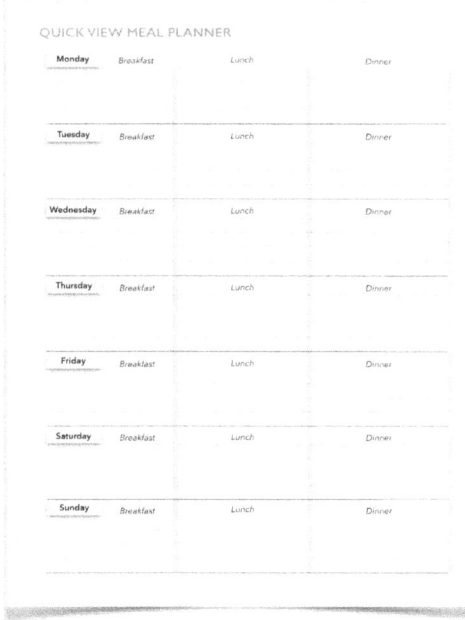

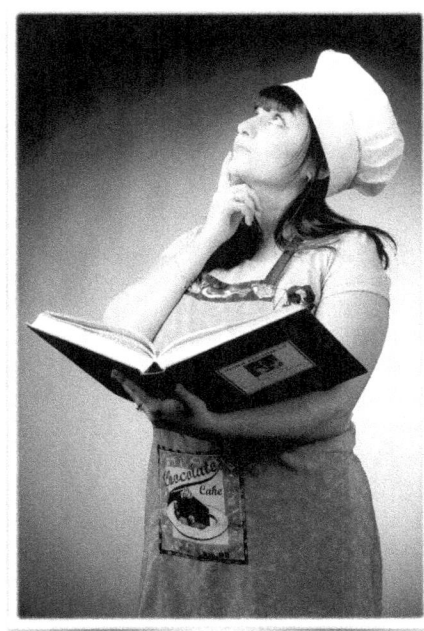

YOUR FOOD JOURNAL PAGE EXPLAINED

Your food journal page has been cleverly worked out and designed to make recording your foods, beverages and calculations super easy.

1. *Why 3 Columns*

2. *Ticks/Beverages*

Monday

BREAKFAST & Morning   *Calories*   **LUNCH** & Afternoon   *Calories*   **DINNER** & Evening   *Calories*

7. *Calorie Goals and Actual*

6. *Drink Totals*

5. *Fruit & Veg*

4. *Mood Tracker*

3. *Steps & Floors*

Morning Calorie Totals

Eve. Calorie Tota

Healthy Options   Slept Well   Steps   Floors

Calorie Goal

Total

Goal   Goal

Actual   A + B + C   Actual

Your Five a Day   Well-Being   Actual   Actual

Everything you need is on one organised page. See the markers above and opposite page numbers for full instructions on how to get the best out of your day!

▷ THREE COLUMNS

1. Why are there three calorie columns, one for breakfast & morning, lunch & afternoon and one for dinner and evening? There is a good answer, read about it on Page **24**

▷ TICKS & BEVERAGES

2. Ticks and Beverages. Place a tick in the blue column each and every time you have a beverage, whether it is coffee, tea or refreshing cold drink.
Read why on Page **26**

▷ STEPS & FLOORS

3. Steps and floors are a great way to burn extra calories. Have a goal and try to hit it everyday! Using a sports watch is a great way to keep you on track.
Details on Page **28**

▷ WELL-BEING

4. Use these tick boxes to monitor your mood. Well-being and sleep are very important! The right mood everyday will result in more weight loss.
More info on Page **25**

▷ FIVE A DAY

5. Track your day's healthy options. Fruit and Vegetables. Five a day is a must, but more is better. Are you getting enough?   Record your daily totals!

▷ REDUCE YOUR BEVERAGES

6. Beverages equal calories and sometimes we drink because of habit and not hydration. Reduce your beverages over time with the Goals and Actual box.
See Page **27**

▷ YOUR DAILY CALORIE GOAL

7. One of the most important boxes on the page. Your daily Calorie allowance or goal and your actual calories! Decide on slow pace or quicker pace! Play around with it so you lose weight, and at the same time feel content!

WHY THREE COLUMNS? ▶

Having three columns will make your life really easy and organised.
Three columns allow you to see at a glance your calorie totals for each section of the day, Morning, Afternoon & Evening, and with this information you can perform some handy calculations. Your calculations allow you to do some "Beneficial Calorie Juggling".

Use the information to juggle and alter your calorie intake. Because you know your daily calorie allowance and the diary page is divided into three sections, you can really juggle around your day's eating. At a glance you can see what calories you had for breakfast allowing you to pre-plan the rest of the day with ease. More snacks or larger lunch, or smaller lunch and more for the evening. Three columns puts you in control.

It's Dinner time, what can I have? Because you know your morning and afternoon totals, you can plan your evening meal better and maximize your meal's calorie value. Simply select a meal from your "Set Menu Pages" that match your available calories left for the day!

You can really play around with this! And I am sure you now see the benefits for three columns and three calorie totals. It's just a better way to be organised.

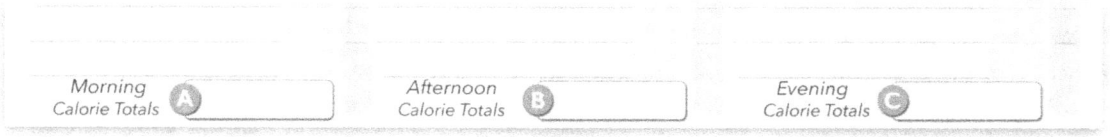

When you know how many calories you have had in the morning and afternoon, you can plan your evening meal to what suits you best! (Maybe your favourite juicy burger - Set menu No.5)

Or work it the other way round, if you have a knockout morning, you can work out a lower calorie evening meal. (Maybe your low Calorie Chicken salad? - Set Menu No.7)

It all works beautifully with your Set Menus for any part of the day. Play around with it - it works - and works well... !

YOUR WELL-BEING

I personally believe that the key to successful dieting and fitness is your mind set. You are about to reduce your calorie intake and increase your activity and we don't want your body, or you, to feel miserable about it.

Very shortly, together we are going to work out your new daily calorie allowance, and this will be your Calorie Goal figure for your diary page. Now, I don't know you personally, I don't know your current weight, body shape, nor do I know your current levels of fitness, stamina and flexibility. So getting that figure spot on straight away may be a little challenging - but not impossible!

Your goal is to get the correct amount of calories in to feel satisfied, lose weight, feel energised and good about yourself at the same time.

So, to help you on the way and ensure you are not getting too much or not enough, I have built in a little 1-5 energy meter on your diary page.
It's very important that you tick this everyday honestly to "How you're feeling". It's an energy meter and not a mood meter! (So don't select a low number because you didn't win the lottery last night).

If you're getting the right amount of calories to keep you satisfied and losing weight at the same time, your daily calories allowance calculations are near spot on. You should be able to place a tick in the 4 to 5 range everyday (Feeling good) and be losing a healthy steady weight!

If the calculations are off and you are not getting enough calories, you will be losing weight, but your body will not be feeling happy about it! Your sleeping patterns may also be affected, making things even worse.

You will no longer feel energised, you will feel tired & irritable (Daily tick ranging between 1 - 3). While in this state, you may be happy with your weight loss - Your body will not be happy with you! And in the end, your body will fight back and it will win!

If you are still getting too many calories, you will soon know about this because: You will not lose any weight! As you progress through the weeks and months, you will have to alter your calorie intake from time to time, so keep ticking these boxes and keep a close eye on them

TICKS & BEVERAGES ▶

Your beverages are just as important as your meals. Lots of people forget that beverages contain calories, or simply say "They don't count", however, they do!

Some people drink more beverages than others. This may be a work environment factor or simply drinking becomes more of a habit rather than a need.

If we all took in fluids for our needs only, we would only drink water. This would be a good thing, but we don't drink to simply nourish and hydrate our bodies anymore, we drink for flavour, enjoyment and to socialise.

Beverages taste nice and supply us with that little boost or kick we're looking for. The most common hot beverages are, you guessed it, tea, coffee and hot chocolate.

For the younger generation it has to be fizzy drinks or an "Iced Frape - something".

Counting ticks is like counting calories.

27 Calories
+
27 Calories
+
27 Calories

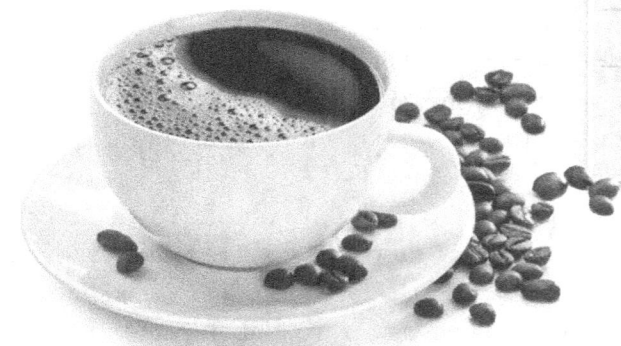

The reason I ask you to place a tick on your diary page each time you have a beverage is so you can see at a glance how many you're having during a single day. **Morning, Afternoon & Evening.**

You may be shocked at the amount you're having, and reducing your beverages alone may be all the difference you're looking for to lose weight - Or it will at least go a long way to help!

Simply looking at the number of ticks on your page may give you a true picture to whether you are just having to many, or too many in one particular part of the day.

You may be able to say to yourself - *No more coffees in the morning*, or I will reduce this by half!

REDUCING BEVERAGES OVER TIME

I suggest for the first week of your diet you stick with you normal number of beverages. Then look back at the end of the week and find the pattern to see how you can realistically reduce the number. You don't want to lose too much of something you love, so start by setting a lower goal target and work it from there.

Set yourself a goal and mark this in your goal target box.

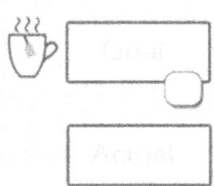

You will be amazed at how reducing your beverages has a marked impact on your weight loss, especially if you have sugar in your tea or coffee.

If you do have sugar in your tea or coffee and you are counting calories, use a measuring spoon instead of a teaspoon. A tea spoon of sugar can vary so much that over time your calorie count can be out by a lot!

Your spoonful may be bigger than mine!

A spoonful of sugar (1tsp 4.2g) is 16 calories. But is your spoonful 16 calories or more? There could be a 5 to 15 calorie difference if your spoonful is heaped. Times this by ten cups and your calorie count is out by as much as 150 calories! (1050 calories per week).

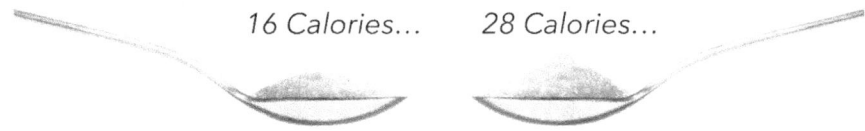

16 Calories...   28 Calories...

It all sounds a little "Picky" but it really does make the difference. When reducing your sugar, don't simply cut it out. Reduce it slowly over a few weeks, using level measuring spoons. This way your taste buds will get used to the small reductions and in a few weeks you can be using the smallest of measuring spoons and your beverage will still taste as sweet. Your beverage will taste just as nice, but you will be getting a fraction of the calories. You may even decide you prefer your drinks with no sugar at all!

YOUR STEPS AND YOUR FLOORS

There's a new personal trainer around and it comes in the form of a fitness watch. Tracking your steps is a great way to lose weight and get fit, and these clever little devices can really push you. Simply look at the watch at any point of the day and see how many steps you have taken and distance travelled.

These smart watches really do push you, and call upon your "Competitive nature" to complete your daily goals. You will find yourself walking a lot more and constantly gauging distances against time.   You will become more conscious about walking and even find yourself going the long way round, simply to add more steps to your counter.

Steps
6,347

Goal ♥
10,000

"Reports and reviews say, that some people pace the living room before going to bed so they can hit their steps goal". That's as good as having your own personal trainer!

There are all types of watches around with varying prices ranges. To be honest you don't need an expensive one, any that track steps is all that is required and you will be able to get yourself one for less than twenty pounds.

The higher the price tag the more functions you can expect to get including, seeing on your watch face who's calling you and text messages.

Walking is sometimes overlooked as a way of exercising. It's probably the easiest form of exercise there is, and will build stamina, burn calories, improve glucose levels and over time reduce your blood pressure. Experts say 10,000 steps is a good number to keep you healthy. Every step counts from around the house, office, shopping and of course "Taking a good walk". Mix it up with different routes, good music or a walking partner.

MORE FLOORS

Although a low to moderate intensity exercise, walking is a great way to burn calories without overdoing it, and it should become part of your daily exercise routine.

Stair walking on the other hand is considered to be a moderate to high intensity exercise and offers even more benefits above walking. Stair walking is an amazing aerobic exercise with the added benefit of toning and strengthening your buttocks and thigh muscles.

Stair walking will burn nearly 3 times more calories per hour than walking on level ground.

Depending on your current body weight & fitness levels, stair walking may tax your energy levels to the max. So don't perform your 10 floors in one session, you can space it out over the day. A simple idea is every time you have to climb a flight of stairs, when you get to the top, turn around, go down and then back up again.

This method will not tax your body too much and you will soon achieve your 10 floors goal everyday.

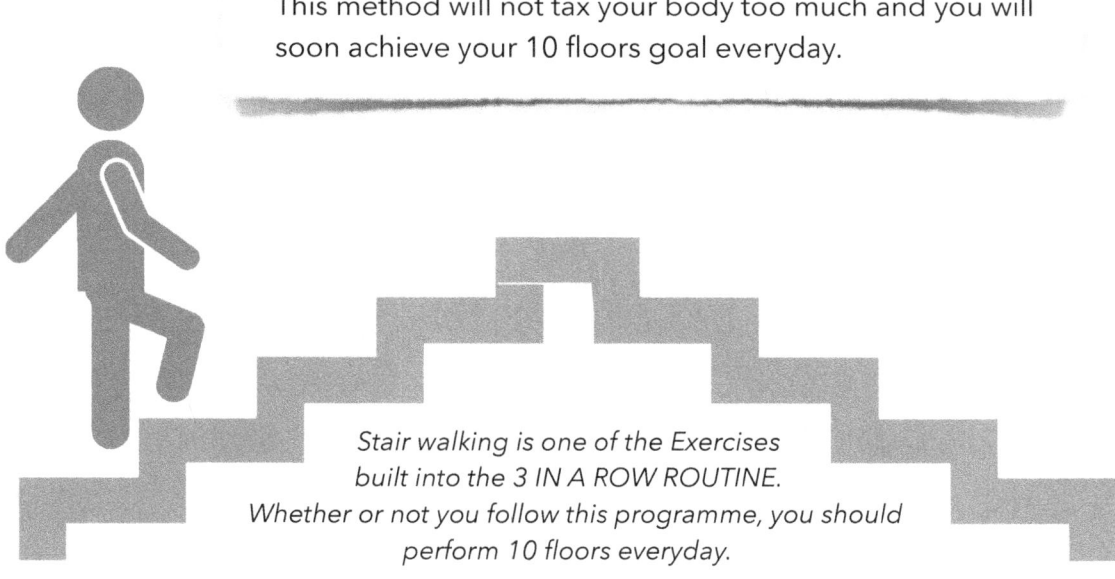

Stair walking is one of the Exercises built into the 3 IN A ROW ROUTINE. Whether or not you follow this programme, you should perform 10 floors everyday.

SECTION 2

A Personal Journey About You and Your Foods!

It is time to get organised!

- About You
- Your Weight Tracker
- Your Measurements Tracker
- Your Notes and Reminders

- Your Shopping Lists
- Your Personal Calorie Library
- Your Personal Set Menus
- Your Meal Planner

- Your Daily Food Journal
- Your Weekly Summary

LETS GO!

Quick Low Calorie Recipes that slot straight into your Set Menus.

Visit our website www.thebodyplanplus.com - Go to Recipes !

Access Password - 232013

▷ NOTES

_____

_____

_____

_____

_____

_____

_____

_____

_____

_____

_____

_____

"The best project you'll ever work on is you"

ABOUT YOU

Have a plan, focus and think! Use this space to write down your plan.
Take some time and don't rush in... Think about it and maybe come back to it later!

▷ **My Goals**   *What are my goals... What motivates me?*

_____

_____

_____

_____

▷ **About Me**   *Write down the things I like, What makes me, me?*

_____

_____

_____

_____

▷ **Why?**   *Write down why I want to make changes in my life!*

_____

_____

_____

_____

▷ **Help!**   *Who can I talk to, and who is going to help me?*

_____

_____

_____

▷ **Relax**   *What am I going to do to relax and unwind?*

▷ **Plan**   *Have something to look forward to! My plans are:*

▷ **Focus**   *My statement to myself, that will keep me focused*

▷ **Finish Line**   *How do you feel after 3 months? What dress size are you in now?*

BODY MEASUREMENTS

When measuring yourself with the measuring tape, the tape should fit snugly against the surface of your skin. It should not press into the skin at any point. When wrapped around you, the measuring tape should be parallel with the floor, and not askew.

When measuring your bust/chest, you'll get the best results if both arms are at your side. You may need assistance for this! When doing your measurements, measure at the same point each time.

Getting the same result, does not mean you haven't lost any weight. Remember your measurements are only guide lines. Measure yourself every other week.

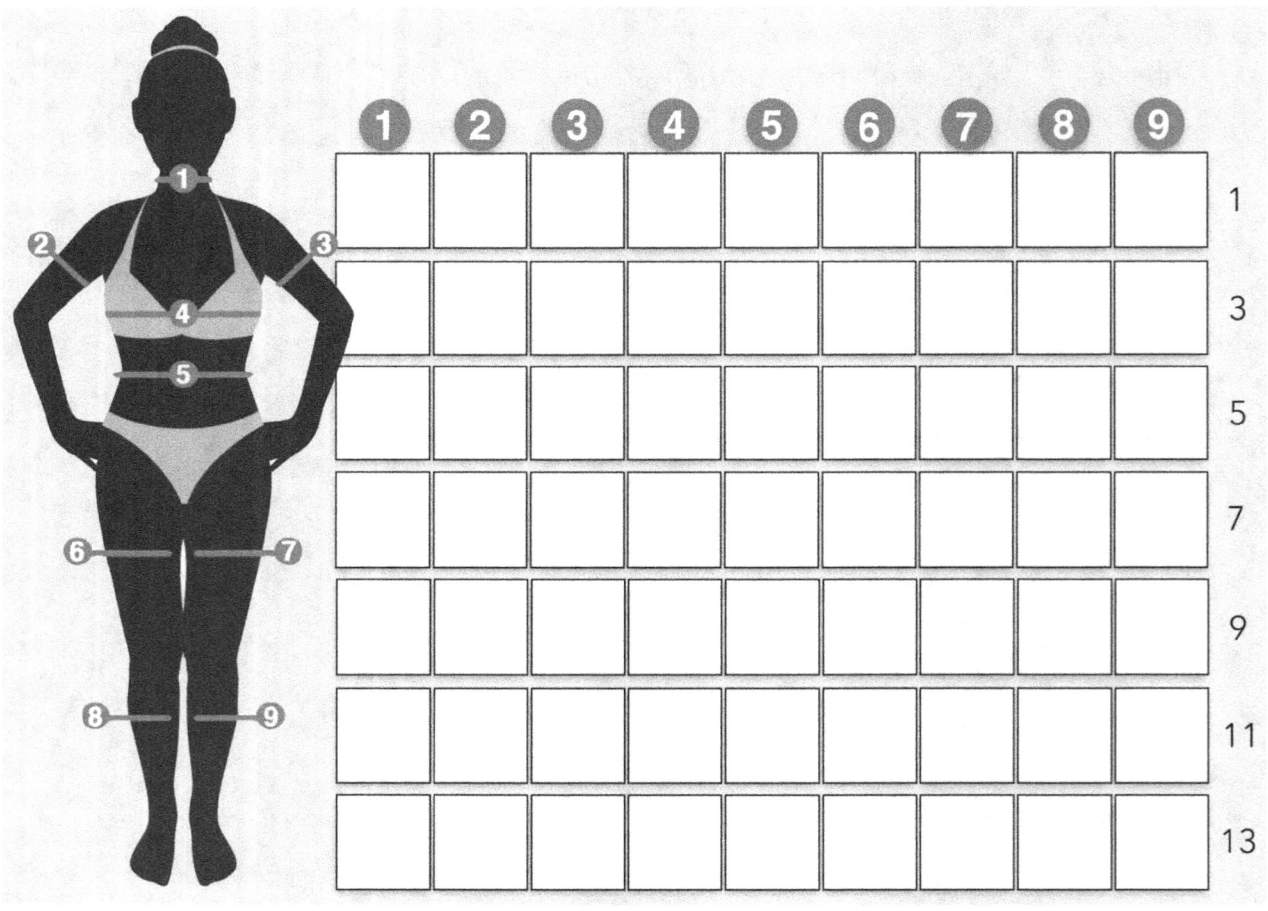

WEIGHT TRACKER & GRAPH

The best time of the day to weigh and measure yourself, is first thing in the morning after you have been to the toilet. Place your scales on an even surface, remove any clothing. Enter Week 1 into the scale box on your graph.

Week **2** Result	Week **3** Result	Week **4** Result	Week **5** Result	Week **6** Result	Week **7** Result
Weigh in **Loss**	**Weigh in** **Loss**	**Weigh in** **Loss**	**Weigh in** **Loss**	**Weigh in** **Loss**	**Weigh in** **Loss**

Week **8** Result	Week **9** Result	Week **10** Result	Week **11** Result	Week **12** Result	Week **13** Result
Weigh in **Loss**	**Weigh in** **Loss**	**Weigh in** **Loss**	**Weigh in** **Loss**	**Weigh in** **Loss**	**Weigh in** **Loss**

lbs
1
2
3
4
5
6
7
8
9
10
11
12
13
14
15
16
17
18
19
20
21
22
23
24
25

Week 1 Week 2 Week 3 Week 4 Week 5 Week 6 Week 7 Week 8 Week 9 Week 10 Week 11 Week 12 Week 13

▷ NOTES

▷ REMINDERS ☑

SHOPPING LIST MUST HAVES

▷ Food item   ▷ Calorie Value   *Low Med High*   *"When I am ready"*
                                                          ▷ Going to Swap for:

▷ Food item   ▷ Calorie Value   *Low Med High*   *"When I am ready"*
▷ Going to Swap for:

SHOPPING LIST MUST HAVES

▷ Food item   ▷ Calorie Value   Low Med High   *"When I am ready"*
▷ Going to Swap for:

Food item	Calorie Value	Low	Med	High	Going to Swap for:
		☐	☐	☐	
		☐	☐	☐	
		☐	☐	☐	
		☐	☐	☐	
		☐	☐	☐	
		☐	☐	☐	
		☐	☐	☐	
		☐	☐	☐	
		☐	☐	☐	
		☐	☐	☐	
		☐	☐	☐	
		☐	☐	☐	
		☐	☐	☐	
		☐	☐	☐	
		☐	☐	☐	
		☐	☐	☐	
		☐	☐	☐	
		☐	☐	☐	
		☐	☐	☐	
		☐	☐	☐	
		☐	☐	☐	
		☐	☐	☐	
		☐	☐	☐	

▷ Food item   ▷ Calorie Value   Low Med High   *"When I am ready"* ▷ Going to Swap for:

BREAKFAST CALORIE LIBRARY

▷ **Food item**　　　　　▷ **Calories** ➡ Per Gram 🔲 Per Portion

		⊗	=	
		⊗	=	
		⊗	=	
		⊗	=	
		⊗	=	
		⊗	=	
		⊗	=	
		⊗	=	
		⊗	=	
		⊗	=	
		⊗	=	
		⊗	=	
		⊗	=	
		⊗	=	
		⊗	=	
		⊗	=	
		⊗	=	

▷ Food item	▷ Calories ⟹ Per Gram	🔲 Per Portion
	✕ ═	
	✕ ═	
	✕ ═	
	✕ ═	
	✕ ═	
	✕ ═	
	✕ ═	
	✕ ═	
	✕ ═	
	✕ ═	
	✕ ═	
	✕ ═	
	✕ ═	
	✕ ═	
	✕ ═	
	✕ ═	
	✕ ═	

LUNCH CALORIE LIBRARY

▷ **Food item**　　　　　　▷ **Calories** ➡ Per Gram 🏋 Per Portion

▷ **Food item**　　　　▷ **Calories** ➡ Per Gram 🏖 Per Portion

	X	=	
	X	=	
	X	=	
	X	=	
	X	=	
	X	=	
	X	=	
	X	=	
	X	=	
	X	=	
	X	=	
	X	=	
	X	=	
	X	=	
	X	=	
	X	=	

DINNER CALORIE LIBRARY

▷ **Food item**　　　　　▷ **Calories** ➡ Per Gram 🔲 Per Portion

(×) (=)

(×) (=)

(×) (=)

(×) (=)

(×) (=)

(×) (=)

(×) (=)

(×) (=)

(×) (=)

(×) (=)

(×) (=)

(×) (=)

(×) (=)

(×) (=)

(×) (=)

(×) (=)

> **Food item**　　　　> **Calories** ➡ Per Gram 🔲 Per Portion

×) =)

×) =)

×) =)

×) =)

×) =)

×) =)

×) =)

×) =)

×) =)

×) =)

×) =)

×) =)

×) =)

×) =)

×) =)

×) =)

×) =)

SNACKS CALORIE LIBRARY

▷ **Food item**　　　　　　　　　▷ **Calories** ➡ Per Gram 🔲 Per Portion

	⊗	⊜
	⊗	⊜
	⊗	⊜
	⊗	⊜
	⊗	⊜
	⊗	⊜
	⊗	⊜
	⊗	⊜
	⊗	⊜
	⊗	⊜
	⊗	⊜
	⊗	⊜
	⊗	⊜
	⊗	⊜
	⊗	⊜
	⊗	⊜
	⊗	⊜

BEVERAGE CALORIE LIBRARY

▷ Beverage	▷ Calories ⟹	Per Gram 🕐	Glass/Cup
		× =	
		× =	
		× =	
		× =	
		× =	
		× =	
		× =	
		× =	
		× =	
		× =	
		× =	
		× =	
		× =	
		× =	
		× =	
		× =	

BREAKFAST SET MENUS

Name | Calories

Menu No.1   Calorie Total

Name | Calories

Menu No.2   Calorie Total

Name | Calories

Menu No.3   Calorie Total

Name | Calories

Menu No.4   Calorie Total

Name | Calories

Menu No.5   Calorie Total

Name | Calories

Menu No.6   Calorie Total

Calories

Name

Menu No.7 **Calorie Total**

Calories

Name

Menu No.8 **Calorie Total**

Calories

Name

Menu No.9 **Calorie Total**

Calories

Name

Menu No.10 **Calorie Total**

Calories

Name

Menu No.11 **Calorie Total**

Calories

Name

Menu No.12 **Calorie Total**

LUNCH SET MENUS

Name _____ Calories

Menu No.1   **Calorie Total** ____

Name _____ Calories

Menu No.2   **Calorie Total** ____

Name _____ Calories

Menu No.3   **Calorie Total** ____

Name _____ Calories

Menu No.4   **Calorie Total** ____

Name _____ Calories

Menu No.5   **Calorie Total** ____

Name _____ Calories

Menu No.6   **Calorie Total** ____

Name

Menu No.7   Calorie Total

Name

Menu No.8   Calorie Total

Name

Menu No.9   Calorie Total

Name

Menu No.10   Calorie Total

Name

Menu No.11   Calorie Total

Name

Menu No.12   Calorie Total

DINNER SET MENUS

Name ⬚ Calories

Menu No.1   **Calorie Total**

Name ⬚ Calories

Menu No.2   **Calorie Total**

Name ⬚ Calories

Menu No.3   **Calorie Total**

Name ⬚ Calories

Menu No.4   **Calorie Total**

Name ⬚ Calories

Menu No.5   **Calorie Total**

Name ⬚ Calories

Menu No.6   **Calorie Total**

Name   Calories

Name   Calories

Menu No.7   **Calorie Total**

Menu No.8   **Calorie Total**

Name   Calories

Name   Calories

Menu No.9   **Calorie Total**

Menu No.10   **Calorie Total**

Name   Calories

Name   Calories

Menu No.11   **Calorie Total**

Menu No.12   **Calorie Total**

▷ WEEK 1 QUICK VIEW MEAL PLANNER

Monday	Breakfast	Lunch	Dinner
Tuesday	Breakfast	Lunch	Dinner
Wednesday	Breakfast	Lunch	Dinner
Thursday	Breakfast	Lunch	Dinner
Friday	Breakfast	Lunch	Dinner
Saturday	Breakfast	Lunch	Dinner
Sunday	Breakfast	Lunch	Dinner

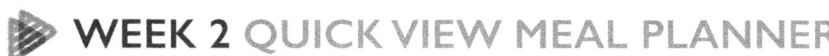

WEEK 2 QUICK VIEW MEAL PLANNER

Monday	*Breakfast*	Lunch	Dinner

Tuesday	*Breakfast*	Lunch	Dinner

Wednesday	*Breakfast*	Lunch	Dinner

Thursday	*Breakfast*	Lunch	Dinner

Friday	*Breakfast*	Lunch	Dinner

Saturday	*Breakfast*	Lunch	Dinner

Sunday	*Breakfast*	*Dinner*	*Lunch*

▶ WEEK 3 QUICK VIEW MEAL PLANNER

Monday	*Breakfast*	*Lunch*	*Dinner*
Tuesday	*Breakfast*	*Lunch*	*Dinner*
Wednesday	*Breakfast*	*Lunch*	*Dinner*
Thursday	*Breakfast*	*Lunch*	*Dinner*
Friday	*Breakfast*	*Lunch*	*Dinner*
Saturday	*Breakfast*	*Lunch*	*Dinner*
Sunday	*Breakfast*	*Lunch*	*Dinner*

WEEK 4 QUICK VIEW MEAL PLANNER

Monday	*Breakfast*	Lunch	Dinner
Tuesday	*Breakfast*	Lunch	Dinner
Wednesday	*Breakfast*	Lunch	Dinner
Thursday	*Breakfast*	Lunch	Dinner
Friday	*Breakfast*	Lunch	Dinner
Saturday	*Breakfast*	Lunch	Dinner
Sunday	*Breakfast*	Dinner	Lunch

▷ WEEK 5 QUICK VIEW MEAL PLANNER

Monday	*Breakfast*	Lunch	Dinner

Tuesday	*Breakfast*	Lunch	Dinner

Wednesday	*Breakfast*	Lunch	Dinner

Thursday	*Breakfast*	Lunch	Dinner

Friday	*Breakfast*	Lunch	Dinner

Saturday	*Breakfast*	Lunch	Dinner

Sunday	*Breakfast*	Lunch	Dinner

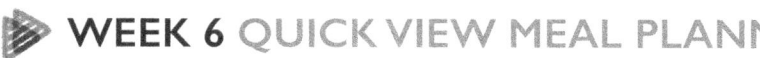

WEEK 6 QUICK VIEW MEAL PLANNER

Monday	*Breakfast*	Lunch	Dinner
Tuesday	*Breakfast*	Lunch	Dinner
Wednesday	*Breakfast*	Lunch	Dinner
Thursday	*Breakfast*	Lunch	Dinner
Friday	*Breakfast*	Lunch	Dinner
Saturday	*Breakfast*	Lunch	Dinner
Sunday	*Breakfast*	Dinner	Lunch

▷ WEEK 7 QUICK VIEW MEAL PLANNER

Monday   *Breakfast*   *Lunch*   *Dinner*

Tuesday   *Breakfast*   *Lunch*   *Dinner*

Wednesday   *Breakfast*   *Lunch*   *Dinner*

Thursday   *Breakfast*   *Lunch*   *Dinner*

Friday   *Breakfast*   *Lunch*   *Dinner*

Saturday   *Breakfast*   *Lunch*   *Dinner*

Sunday   *Breakfast*   *Lunch*   *Dinner*

▶ WEEK 8 QUICK VIEW MEAL PLANNER

Monday	*Breakfast*	Lunch	Dinner

Tuesday	*Breakfast*	Lunch	Dinner

Wednesday	*Breakfast*	Lunch	Dinner

Thursday	*Breakfast*	Lunch	Dinner

Friday	*Breakfast*	Lunch	Dinner

Saturday	*Breakfast*	Lunch	Dinner

Sunday	*Breakfast*	Dinner	Lunch

▶ WEEK 9 QUICK VIEW MEAL PLANNER

Monday	*Breakfast*	*Lunch*	*Dinner*
Tuesday	*Breakfast*	*Lunch*	*Dinner*
Wednesday	*Breakfast*	*Lunch*	*Dinner*
Thursday	*Breakfast*	*Lunch*	*Dinner*
Friday	*Breakfast*	*Lunch*	*Dinner*
Saturday	*Breakfast*	*Lunch*	*Dinner*
Sunday	*Breakfast*	*Lunch*	*Dinner*

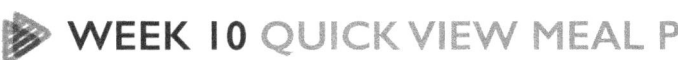

WEEK 10 QUICK VIEW MEAL PLANNER

Monday	*Breakfast*	Lunch	Dinner
Tuesday	*Breakfast*	Lunch	Dinner
Wednesday	*Breakfast*	Lunch	Dinner
Thursday	*Breakfast*	Lunch	Dinner
Friday	*Breakfast*	Lunch	Dinner
Saturday	*Breakfast*	Lunch	Dinner
Sunday	*Breakfast*	Dinner	Lunch

▶ WEEK 11 QUICK VIEW MEAL PLANNER

Monday	*Breakfast*	Lunch	Dinner
Tuesday	*Breakfast*	Lunch	Dinner
Wednesday	*Breakfast*	Lunch	Dinner
Thursday	*Breakfast*	Lunch	Dinner
Friday	*Breakfast*	Lunch	Dinner
Saturday	*Breakfast*	Lunch	Dinner
Sunday	*Breakfast*	Lunch	Dinner

WEEK 12 QUICK VIEW MEAL PLANNER

Monday	Breakfast	Lunch	Dinner

Tuesday	Breakfast	Lunch	Dinner

Wednesday	Breakfast	Lunch	Dinner

Thursday	Breakfast	Lunch	Dinner

Friday	Breakfast	Lunch	Dinner

Saturday	Breakfast	Lunch	Dinner

Sunday	Breakfast	Dinner	Lunch

▷ WEEK 13 QUICK VIEW MEAL PLANNER

Monday   *Breakfast*   Lunch   *Dinner*

Tuesday   *Breakfast*   Lunch   *Dinner*

Wednesday   *Breakfast*   Lunch   *Dinner*

Thursday   *Breakfast*   Lunch   *Dinner*

Friday   *Breakfast*   Lunch   *Dinner*

Saturday   *Breakfast*   Lunch   *Dinner*

Sunday   *Breakfast*   Lunch   *Dinner*

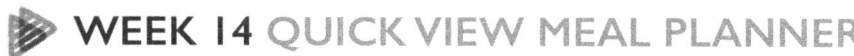

WEEK 14 QUICK VIEW MEAL PLANNER

Monday	*Breakfast*	*Lunch*	*Dinner*
Tuesday	*Breakfast*	*Lunch*	*Dinner*
Wednesday	*Breakfast*	*Lunch*	*Dinner*
Thursday	*Breakfast*	*Lunch*	*Dinner*
Friday	*Breakfast*	*Lunch*	*Dinner*
Saturday	*Breakfast*	*Lunch*	*Dinner*
Sunday	*Breakfast*	*Dinner*	*Lunch*

NOTES

REMINDERS

☑
☐
☐
☐
☐
☐
☐
☐

▷ MONDAY

BREAKFAST *& Morning* | Calories ☕ | **LUNCH** *& Afternoon* | Calories ☕ | **DINNER** *& Evening* | Calories ☕

Morning Calorie Totals (A)

Afternoon Calorie Totals (B)

Evening Calorie Totals (C)

Calorie Goal

(A) + (B) + (C)

Actual

☕

Healthy Options

Your Five a Day

Slept Well
1 z 2 z 3 z 4 z 5 z

Well-Being
1 2 3 4 5

Steps Floors

▷ TUESDAY

BREAKFAST *& Morning* | Calories ☕ | **LUNCH** *& Afternoon* | Calories ☕ | **DINNER** *& Evening* | Calories ☕

Morning Calorie Totals (A)

Afternoon Calorie Totals (B)

Evening Calorie Totals (C)

Calorie Goal

(A) + (B) + (C)

Actual

☕

Healthy Options

Your Five a Day

Slept Well
1 z 2 z 3 z 4 z 5 z

Well-Being
1 2 3 4 5

Steps Floors

▷ WEDNESDAY

BREAKFAST *& Morning*	*Calories* ☕	**LUNCH** *& Afternoon*	*Calories* ☕	**DINNER** *& Evening*	*Calories* ☕

Morning Calorie Totals **A**	*Afternoon Calorie Totals* **B**	*Evening Calorie Totals* **C**

Calorie Goal

Actual Ⓐ + Ⓑ + Ⓒ

☕

Healthy Options

Your Five a Day

Slept Well
① ② ③ ④ ⑤

Well-Being
① ② ③ ④ ⑤

Steps   Floors

▷ THURSDAY

BREAKFAST *& Morning*	*Calories* ☕	**LUNCH** *& Afternoon*	*Calories* ☕	**DINNER** *& Evening*	*Calories* ☕

Morning Calorie Totals **A**	*Afternoon Calorie Totals* **B**	*Evening Calorie Totals* **C**

Calorie Goal

Actual Ⓐ + Ⓑ + Ⓒ

☕

Healthy Options

Your Five a Day

Slept Well
① ② ③ ④ ⑤

Well-Being
① ② ③ ④ ⑤

Steps   Floors

▷ FRIDAY

BREAKFAST *& Morning*   *Calories* ☕   **LUNCH** *& Afternoon*   *Calories* ☕   **DINNER** *& Evening*   *Calories* ☕

Morning
Calorie Totals **A**

Calorie Goal

A + **B** + **C**

Actual

Afternoon
Calorie Totals **B**

☕

Healthy Options

Your Five a Day

Evening
Calorie Totals **C**

Slept Well
1 z 2 z 3 z 4 z 5 z

Well-Being
1 2 3 4 5

Steps   Floors

▷ SATURDAY

BREAKFAST *& Morning*   *Calories* ☕   **LUNCH** *& Afternoon*   *Calories* ☕   **DINNER** *& Evening*   *Calories* ☕

Morning
Calorie Totals **A**

Calorie Goal

A + **B** + **C**

Actual

Afternoon
Calorie Totals **B**

☕

Healthy Options

Your Five a Day

Evening
Calorie Totals **C**

Slept Well
1 z 2 z 3 z 4 z 5 z

Well-Being
1 2 3 4 5

Steps   Floors

▷ SUNDAY

BREAKFAST *& Morning* | *Calories* | ☕ | **LUNCH** *& Afternoon* | *Calories* | ☕ | **DINNER** *& Evening* | *Calories* | ☕

| Morning Calorie Totals | Ⓐ | | | Afternoon Calorie Totals | Ⓑ | | | Evening Calorie Totals | Ⓒ | |

Calorie Goal

☕

Actual   Ⓐ + Ⓑ + Ⓒ

Healthy Options

Your Five a Day

Slept Well
1 2 3 4 5

Well-Being
1 2 3 4 5

Steps   Floors

▷ WEEK 1 SUMMARY

	Mon	Tue	Wed	Thur	Fri	Sat	Sun

Weekly Calorie Totals

Weekly Beverage (No.of ticks) Totals

Your Vegetable Weekly Totals

Your Fruit Weekly Totals

Your Steps & Floors

35
30
25
15
10
5

Mon Tue Wed Thur Fri Sat Sun

10k
9k
8k
7k
6k
5k
4k

Mon Tue Wed Thur Fri Sat Sun

▷ MONDAY

BREAKFAST *& Morning* Calories ☕ **LUNCH** *& Afternoon* Calories ☕ **DINNER** *& Evening* Calories ☕

Morning Calorie Totals (A) _____

Afternoon Calorie Totals (B) _____

Evening Calorie Totals (C) _____

Calorie Goal _____

☕ _____

Actual (A) + (B) + (C) _____

_____

Healthy Options
🥕 🥕 🥕 🥕

Your Five a Day
🍎 🍎 🍎 🍎

Slept Well
1z 2z 3z 4z 5z

Well-Being
1 2 3 4 5

Steps Floors

____ ____

____ ____

▷ TUESDAY

BREAKFAST *& Morning* Calories ☕ **LUNCH** *& Afternoon* Calories ☕ **DINNER** *& Evening* Calories ☕

Morning Calorie Totals (A) _____

Afternoon Calorie Totals (B) _____

Evening Calorie Totals (C) _____

Calorie Goal _____

☕ _____

Actual (A) + (B) + (C) _____

_____

Healthy Options
🥕 🥕 🥕 🥕

Your Five a Day
🍎 🍎 🍎 🍎

Slept Well
1z 2z 3z 4z 5z

Well-Being
1 2 3 4 5

Steps Floors

____ ____

____ ____

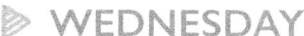 WEDNESDAY

BREAKFAST *& Morning* *Calories* | **LUNCH** *& Afternoon* *Calories* | **DINNER** *& Evening* *Calories*

Morning Calorie Totals (A)

Afternoon Calorie Totals (B)

Evening Calorie Totals (C)

Calorie Goal

Actual   (A) + (B) + (C)

Healthy Options

Your Five a Day

Slept Well
1 z 2 z 3 z 4 z 5 z

Well-Being
1 2 3 4 5

Steps   Floors

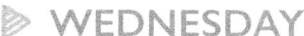 THURSDAY

BREAKFAST *& Morning* *Calories* | **LUNCH** *& Afternoon* *Calories* | **DINNER** *& Evening* *Calories*

Morning Calorie Totals (A)

Afternoon Calorie Totals (B)

Evening Calorie Totals (C)

Calorie Goal

Actual   (A) + (B) + (C)

Healthy Options

Your Five a Day

Slept Well
1 z 2 z 3 z 4 z 5 z

Well-Being
1 2 3 4 5

Steps   Floors

▷ FRIDAY

BREAKFAST *& Morning* *Calories* ☕ **LUNCH** *& Afternoon* *Calories* ☕ **DINNER** *& Evening* *Calories* ☕

Morning
Calorie Totals (A)

Afternoon
Calorie Totals (B)

Evening
Calorie Totals (C)

Calorie Goal

☕

Healthy Options

Slept Well
①z ②z ③z ④z ⑤z

Steps   Floors

Actual (A) + (B) + (C)

Your Five a Day

Well-Being
① ② ③ ④ ⑤

▷ SATURDAY

BREAKFAST *& Morning* *Calories* ☕ **LUNCH** *& Afternoon* *Calories* ☕ **DINNER** *& Evening* *Calories* ☕

Morning
Calorie Totals (A)

Afternoon
Calorie Totals (B)

Evening
Calorie Totals (C)

Calorie Goal

☕

Healthy Options

Slept Well
①z ②z ③z ④z ⑤z

Steps   Floors

Actual (A) + (B) + (C)

Your Five a Day

Well-Being
① ② ③ ④ ⑤

▷ SUNDAY

BREAKFAST *& Morning* *Calories* ☕ **LUNCH** *& Afternoon* *Calories* ☕ **DINNER** *& Evening* *Calories* ☕

Morning Calorie Totals	Ⓐ		Afternoon Calorie Totals	Ⓑ		Evening Calorie Totals	Ⓒ	

Calorie Goal

☕

Actual Ⓐ + Ⓑ + Ⓒ

Healthy Options

Your Five a Day

Slept Well ①z ②z ③z ④z ⑤z

Well-Being ① ② ③ ④ ⑤

Steps   Floors

▷ WEEK 2 SUMMARY

	Mon	Tue	Wed	Thur	Fri	Sat	Sun

🔥 *Weekly Calorie Totals*

☕ *Weekly Beverage (No.of ticks) Totals*

🥕 *Your Vegetable Weekly Totals*

🍎 *Your Fruit Weekly Totals*

Your Steps & Floors

35
30
25
15
10
5

Mon Tue Wed Thur Fri Sat Sun

10k
9k
8k
7k
6k
5k
4k

Mon Tue Wed Thur Fri Sat Sun

▷ MONDAY

BREAKFAST *& Morning*   *Calories*   ☕   **LUNCH** *& Afternoon*   *Calories*   ☕   **DINNER** *& Evening*   *Calories*   ☕

Morning Calorie Totals (A) _____   *Afternoon Calorie Totals* (B) _____   *Evening Calorie Totals* (C) _____

Calorie Goal _____

Actual (A) + (B) + (C)

☕ _____

_____

Healthy Options
🥕 🥕 🥕 🥕

Your Five a Day
🍎 🍎 🍎 🍎

Slept Well
1z 2z 3z 4z 5z

Well-Being
1 2 3 4 5

Steps   Floors
_____   _____
_____   _____

▷ TUESDAY

BREAKFAST *& Morning*   *Calories*   ☕   **LUNCH** *& Afternoon*   *Calories*   ☕   **DINNER** *& Evening*   *Calories*   ☕

Morning Calorie Totals (A) _____   *Afternoon Calorie Totals* (B) _____   *Evening Calorie Totals* (C) _____

Calorie Goal _____

Actual (A) + (B) + (C)

☕ _____

_____

Healthy Options
🥕 🥕 🥕 🥕

Your Five a Day
🍎 🍎 🍎 🍎

Slept Well
1z 2z 3z 4z 5z

Well-Being
1 2 3 4 5

Steps   Floors
_____   _____
_____   _____

WEDNESDAY

BREAKFAST *& Morning* *Calories* | **LUNCH** *& Afternoon* *Calories* | **DINNER** *& Evening* *Calories*

Morning Calorie Totals (A)

Afternoon Calorie Totals (B)

Evening Calorie Totals (C)

Calorie Goal

Actual (A) + (B) + (C)

Healthy Options

Your Five a Day

Slept Well
1 2 3 4 5

Well-Being
1 2 3 4 5

Steps Floors

THURSDAY

BREAKFAST *& Morning* *Calories* | **LUNCH** *& Afternoon* *Calories* | **DINNER** *& Evening* *Calories*

Morning Calorie Totals (A)

Afternoon Calorie Totals (B)

Evening Calorie Totals (C)

Calorie Goal

Actual (A) + (B) + (C)

Healthy Options

Your Five a Day

Slept Well
1 2 3 4 5

Well-Being
1 2 3 4 5

Steps Floors

FRIDAY

BREAKFAST *& Morning* — *Calories* ☕ | **LUNCH** *& Afternoon* — *Calories* ☕ | **DINNER** *& Evening* — *Calories* ☕

Morning **A** Calorie Totals

Calorie Goal

Actual   **A** + **B** + **C**

Afternoon **B** Calorie Totals

☕

Healthy Options

Your Five a Day

Slept Well
1 z 2 z 3 z 4 z 5 z

Well-Being
1 2 3 4 5

Evening **C** Calorie Totals

Steps   Floors

SATURDAY

BREAKFAST *& Morning* — *Calories* ☕ | **LUNCH** *& Afternoon* — *Calories* ☕ | **DINNER** *& Evening* — *Calories* ☕

Morning **A** Calorie Totals

Calorie Goal

Actual   **A** + **B** + **C**

Afternoon **B** Calorie Totals

☕

Healthy Options

Your Five a Day

Slept Well
1 z 2 z 3 z 4 z 5 z

Well-Being
1 2 3 4 5

Evening **C** Calorie Totals

Steps   Floors

▷ SUNDAY

BREAKFAST *& Morning*	Calories	**LUNCH** *& Afternoon*	Calories	**DINNER** *& Evening*	Calories

Morning Calorie Totals Ⓐ

Calorie Goal

Actual Ⓐ + Ⓑ + Ⓒ

Afternoon Calorie Totals Ⓑ

Evening Calorie Totals Ⓒ

Healthy Options

Your Five a Day

Slept Well
1 2 3 4 5

Well-Being
1 2 3 4 5

Steps **Floors**

▷ WEEK 3 SUMMARY

	Mon	Tue	Wed	Thur	Fri	Sat	Sun
Weekly Calorie Totals							
Weekly Beverage (No.of ticks) Totals							
Your Vegetable Weekly Totals							
Your Fruit Weekly Totals							

Your Steps & Floors

35
30
25
15
10
5

Mon Tue Wed Thur Fri Sat Sun

10k
9k
8k
7k
6k
5k
4k

Mon Tue Wed Thur Fri Sat Sun

▶ MONDAY

BREAKFAST *& Morning*   *Calories*   **LUNCH** *& Afternoon*   *Calories*   **DINNER** *& Evening*   *Calories*

Morning
Calorie Totals   Ⓐ

Afternoon
Calorie Totals   Ⓑ

Evening
Calorie Totals   Ⓒ

Calorie Goal

Ⓐ + Ⓑ + Ⓒ

Actual

Healthy Options

Your Five a Day

Slept Well

1z 2z 3z 4z 5z

Well-Being

1 2 3 4 5

Steps   Floors

▶ TUESDAY

BREAKFAST *& Morning*   *Calories*   **LUNCH** *& Afternoon*   *Calories*   **DINNER** *& Evening*   *Calories*

Morning
Calorie Totals   Ⓐ

Afternoon
Calorie Totals   Ⓑ

Evening
Calorie Totals   Ⓒ

Calorie Goal

Ⓐ + Ⓑ + Ⓒ

Actual

Healthy Options

Your Five a Day

Slept Well

1z 2z 3z 4z 5z

Well-Being

1 2 3 4 5

Steps   Floors

▷ WEDNESDAY

BREAKFAST *& Morning* *Calories* ☕ **LUNCH** *& Afternoon* *Calories* ☕ **DINNER** *& Evening* *Calories* ☕

Morning Calorie Totals Ⓐ

Calorie Goal

Actual   Ⓐ + Ⓑ + Ⓒ

Afternoon Calorie Totals Ⓑ

☕

Healthy Options

Your Five a Day

Slept Well
① ② ③ ④ ⑤
z z z z z

Well-Being
① ② ③ ④ ⑤

Evening Calorie Totals Ⓒ

Steps   Floors

▷ THURSDAY

BREAKFAST *& Morning* *Calories* ☕ **LUNCH** *& Afternoon* *Calories* ☕ **DINNER** *& Evening* *Calories* ☕

Morning Calorie Totals Ⓐ

Calorie Goal

Actual   Ⓐ + Ⓑ + Ⓒ

Afternoon Calorie Totals Ⓑ

☕

Healthy Options

Your Five a Day

Slept Well
① ② ③ ④ ⑤
z z z z z

Well-Being
① ② ③ ④ ⑤

Evening Calorie Totals Ⓒ

Steps   Floors

▷ FRIDAY

BREAKFAST & Morning	Calories ☕	LUNCH & Afternoon	Calories ☕	DINNER & Evening	Calories ☕

Morning Calorie Totals **A** _____

Afternoon Calorie Totals **B** _____

Evening Calorie Totals **C** _____

Calorie Goal _____

☕ _____

Actual **A** + **B** + **C** _____

Healthy Options
🥕 🥕 🥕 🥕

Your Five a Day
🍎 🍎 🍎 🍎

Slept Well
1 z 2 z 3 z 4 z 5 z

Well-Being
1 😖 2 😣 3 😐 4 🙂 5 😊

Steps **Floors**

▷ SATURDAY

BREAKFAST & Morning	Calories ☕	LUNCH & Afternoon	Calories ☕	DINNER & Evening	Calories ☕

Morning Calorie Totals **A** _____

Afternoon Calorie Totals **B** _____

Evening Calorie Totals **C** _____

Calorie Goal _____

☕ _____

Actual **A** + **B** + **C** _____

Healthy Options
🥕 🥕 🥕 🥕

Your Five a Day
🍎 🍎 🍎 🍎

Slept Well
1 z 2 z 3 z 4 z 5 z

Well-Being
1 😖 2 😣 3 😐 4 🙂 5 😊

Steps **Floors**

▷ SUNDAY

BREAKFAST *& Morning* *Calories* ☕   **LUNCH** *& Afternoon* *Calories* ☕   **DINNER** *& Evening* *Calories* ☕

Morning Calorie Totals (A)

Afternoon Calorie Totals (B)

Evening Calorie Totals (C)

Calorie Goal

Actual (A) + (B) + (C)

☕

Healthy Options

Your Five a Day

Slept Well
1 2 3 4 5

Well-Being
1 2 3 4 5

Steps Floors

▷ WEEK 4 SUMMARY

	Mon	Tue	Wed	Thur	Fri	Sat	Sun

Weekly Calorie Totals

☕ *Weekly Beverage (No.of ticks) Totals*

🥕 *Your Vegetable Weekly Totals*

🍎 *Your Fruit Weekly Totals*

Your Steps & Floors

35
30
25
15
10
5

Mon Tue Wed Thur Fri Sat Sun

10k
9k
8k
7k
6k
5k
4k

Mon Tue Wed Thur Fri Sat Sun

▷ MONDAY

BREAKFAST *& Morning* *Calories* ☕   **LUNCH** *& Afternoon* *Calories* ☕   **DINNER** *& Evening* *Calories* ☕

Morning **A**
Calorie Totals

Afternoon **B**
Calorie Totals

Evening **C**
Calorie Totals

Calorie Goal

☕

Healthy Options

Slept Well
1 z 2 z 3 z 4 z 5 z

Steps **Floors**

Actual Ⓐ + Ⓑ + Ⓒ

Your Five a Day

Well-Being
1 2 3 4 5

▷ TUESDAY

BREAKFAST *& Morning* *Calories* ☕   **LUNCH** *& Afternoon* *Calories* ☕   **DINNER** *& Evening* *Calories* ☕

Morning **A**
Calorie Totals

Afternoon **B**
Calorie Totals

Evening **C**
Calorie Totals

Calorie Goal

☕

Healthy Options

Slept Well
1 z 2 z 3 z 4 z 5 z

Steps **Floors**

Actual Ⓐ + Ⓑ + Ⓒ

Your Five a Day

Well-Being
1 2 3 4 5

WEDNESDAY

BREAKFAST *& Morning* *Calories* **LUNCH** *& Afternoon* *Calories* **DINNER** *& Evening* *Calories*

Morning Calorie Totals **A**

Afternoon Calorie Totals **B**

Evening Calorie Totals **C**

Calorie Goal

Actual **A** + **B** + **C**

Healthy Options

Your Five a Day

Slept Well
1 z 2 z 3 z 4 z 5 z

Well-Being
1 2 3 4 5

Steps Floors

THURSDAY

BREAKFAST *& Morning* *Calories* **LUNCH** *& Afternoon* *Calories* **DINNER** *& Evening* *Calories*

Morning Calorie Totals **A**

Afternoon Calorie Totals **B**

Evening Calorie Totals **C**

Calorie Goal

Actual **A** + **B** + **C**

Healthy Options

Your Five a Day

Slept Well
1 z 2 z 3 z 4 z 5 z

Well-Being
1 2 3 4 5

Steps Floors

▷ FRIDAY

BREAKFAST *& Morning*   *Calories* ☕

LUNCH *& Afternoon*   *Calories* ☕

DINNER *& Evening*   *Calories* ☕

Morning
Calorie Totals (A)

Afternoon
Calorie Totals (B)

Evening
Calorie Totals (C)

Calorie Goal

☕

Healthy Options

Slept Well
1 z 2 z 3 z 4 z 5 z

Steps   Floors

Actual   (A) + (B) + (C)

Your Five a Day

Well-Being
1 2 3 4 5

▷ SATURDAY

BREAKFAST *& Morning*   *Calories* ☕

LUNCH *& Afternoon*   *Calories* ☕

DINNER *& Evening*   *Calories* ☕

Morning
Calorie Totals (A)

Afternoon
Calorie Totals (B)

Evening
Calorie Totals (C)

Calorie Goal

☕

Healthy Options

Slept Well
1 z 2 z 3 z 4 z 5 z

Steps   Floors

Actual   (A) + (B) + (C)

Your Five a Day

Well-Being
1 2 3 4 5

BREAKFAST *& Morning* *Calories* ☕   **LUNCH** *& Afternoon* *Calories* ☕   **DINNER** *& Evening* *Calories* ☕

Morning
Calorie Totals (A)

Afternoon
Calorie Totals (B)

Evening
Calorie Totals (C)

Calorie Goal

☕

Healthy Options

Slept Well

Steps   Floors

Ⓐ + Ⓑ + Ⓒ

Actual

Your Five a Day

Well-Being

▷ WEEK 5 SUMMARY

	Mon	Tue	Wed	Thur	Fri	Sat	Sun
🔥			*Weekly Calorie Totals*				
☕			*Weekly Beverage (No.of ticks) Totals*				
🥕			*Your Vegetable Weekly Totals*				
🍎			*Your Fruit Weekly Totals*				

Your Steps & Floors

35
30
25
15
10
5

Mon   Tue   Wed   Thur   Fri   Sat   Sun

10k
9k
8k
7k
6k
5k
4k

Mon   Tue   Wed   Thur   Fri   Sat   Sun

▷ MONDAY

BREAKFAST *& Morning* *Calories* ☕   **LUNCH** *& Afternoon* *Calories* ☕   **DINNER** *& Evening* *Calories* ☕

Morning
Calorie Totals (A)

Afternoon
Calorie Totals (B)

Evening
Calorie Totals (C)

Calorie Goal

☕

Healthy Options

Slept Well
1 z 2 z 3 z 4 z 5 z

Steps   Floors

Actual   (A) + (B) + (C)

Your Five a Day

Well-Being
1 2 3 4 5

▷ TUESDAY

BREAKFAST *& Morning* *Calories* ☕   **LUNCH** *& Afternoon* *Calories* ☕   **DINNER** *& Evening* *Calories* ☕

Morning
Calorie Totals (A)

Afternoon
Calorie Totals (B)

Evening
Calorie Totals (C)

Calorie Goal

☕

Healthy Options

Slept Well
1 z 2 z 3 z 4 z 5 z

Steps   Floors

Actual   (A) + (B) + (C)

Your Five a Day

Well-Being
1 2 3 4 5

▷ WEDNESDAY

BREAKFAST *& Morning* Calories ☕ **LUNCH** *& Afternoon* Calories ☕ **DINNER** *& Evening* Calories ☕

Morning Calorie Totals Ⓐ

Calorie Goal

Actual Ⓐ + Ⓑ + Ⓒ

Afternoon Calorie Totals Ⓑ

☕

Evening Calorie Totals Ⓒ

Healthy Options

Your Five a Day

Slept Well
1 z 2 z 3 z 4 z 5 z

Well-Being
1 2 3 4 5

Steps Floors

▷ THURSDAY

BREAKFAST *& Morning* Calories ☕ **LUNCH** *& Afternoon* Calories ☕ **DINNER** *& Evening* Calories ☕

Morning Calorie Totals Ⓐ

Calorie Goal

Actual Ⓐ + Ⓑ + Ⓒ

Afternoon Calorie Totals Ⓑ

☕

Evening Calorie Totals Ⓒ

Healthy Options

Your Five a Day

Slept Well
1 z 2 z 3 z 4 z 5 z

Well-Being
1 2 3 4 5

Steps Floors

FRIDAY

BREAKFAST *& Morning* *Calories*

LUNCH *& Afternoon* *Calories*

DINNER *& Evening* *Calories*

Morning Calorie Totals **A**

Calorie Goal

Actual **A + B + C**

Afternoon Calorie Totals **B**

Healthy Options

Your Five a Day

Slept Well
1 2 3 4 5

Well-Being
1 2 3 4 5

Evening Calorie Totals **C**

Steps   Floors

SATURDAY

BREAKFAST *& Morning* *Calories*

LUNCH *& Afternoon* *Calories*

DINNER *& Evening* *Calories*

Morning Calorie Totals **A**

Calorie Goal

Actual **A + B + C**

Afternoon Calorie Totals **B**

Healthy Options

Your Five a Day

Slept Well
1 2 3 4 5

Well-Being
1 2 3 4 5

Evening Calorie Totals **C**

Steps   Floors

▷ SUNDAY

BREAKFAST *& Morning*   *Calories*   ☕   **LUNCH** *& Afternoon*   *Calories*   ☕   **DINNER** *& Evening*   *Calories*   ☕

Morning Calorie Totals (A)	*Afternoon Calorie Totals* (B)	*Evening Calorie Totals* (C)

Calorie Goal

Actual   (A) + (B) + (C)

☕

Healthy Options   **Slept Well**   **Steps**   **Floors**

Your Five a Day   **Well-Being**

▷ WEEK 6 SUMMARY

	Mon	Tue	Wed	Thur	Fri	Sat	Sun

Weekly Calorie Totals

Your Steps & Floors

35
30
25
15
10
5

Mon Tue Wed Thur Fri Sat Sun

☕ *Weekly Beverage (No. of ticks) Totals*

10k
9k
8k
7k
6k
5k
4k

Your Vegetable Weekly Totals

Your Fruit Weekly Totals

Mon Tue Wed Thur Fri Sat Sun

▷ MONDAY

BREAKFAST *& Morning* Calories

LUNCH *& Afternoon* Calories

DINNER *& Evening* Calories

Morning Calorie Totals Ⓐ

Afternoon Calorie Totals Ⓑ

Evening Calorie Totals Ⓒ

Calorie Goal

Actual Ⓐ + Ⓑ + Ⓒ

Healthy Options

Your Five a Day

Slept Well
1 z 2 z 3 z 4 z 5 z

Well-Being
1 2 3 4 5

Steps   Floors

▷ TUESDAY

BREAKFAST *& Morning* Calories

LUNCH *& Afternoon* Calories

DINNER *& Evening* Calories

Morning Calorie Totals Ⓐ

Afternoon Calorie Totals Ⓑ

Evening Calorie Totals Ⓒ

Calorie Goal

Actual Ⓐ + Ⓑ + Ⓒ

Healthy Options

Your Five a Day

Slept Well
1 z 2 z 3 z 4 z 5 z

Well-Being
1 2 3 4 5

Steps   Floors

▷ WEDNESDAY

BREAKFAST & *Morning*　*Calories* ☕　**LUNCH** & *Afternoon*　*Calories* ☕　**DINNER** & *Evening*　*Calories* ☕

Morning Calorie Totals (A)

Afternoon Calorie Totals (B)

Evening Calorie Totals (C)

Calorie Goal

☕

Healthy Options

Slept Well
1 z 2 z 3 z 4 z 5 z

Steps　Floors

Actual
(A) + (B) + (C)

Your Five a Day

Well-Being
1 2 3 4 5

▷ THURSDAY

BREAKFAST & *Morning*　*Calories* ☕　**LUNCH** & *Afternoon*　*Calories* ☕　**DINNER** & *Evening*　*Calories* ☕

Morning Calorie Totals (A)

Afternoon Calorie Totals (B)

Evening Calorie Totals (C)

Calorie Goal

☕

Healthy Options

Slept Well
1 z 2 z 3 z 4 z 5 z

Steps　Floors

Actual
(A) + (B) + (C)

Your Five a Day

Well-Being
1 2 3 4 5

▷ FRIDAY

BREAKFAST & *Morning*   *Calories*   **LUNCH** & *Afternoon*   *Calories*   **DINNER** & *Evening*   *Calories*

Morning (A)
Calorie Totals

Afternoon (B)
Calorie Totals

Evening (C)
Calorie Totals

Calorie Goal

Actual   (A) + (B) + (C)

Healthy Options

Your Five a Day

Slept Well
1 z 2 z 3 z 4 z 5 z

Well-Being
1 2 3 4 5

Steps   Floors

▷ SATURDAY

BREAKFAST & *Morning*   *Calories*   **LUNCH** & *Afternoon*   *Calories*   **DINNER** & *Evening*   *Calories*

Morning (A)
Calorie Totals

Afternoon (B)
Calorie Totals

Evening (C)
Calorie Totals

Calorie Goal

Actual   (A) + (B) + (C)

Healthy Options

Your Five a Day

Slept Well
1 z 2 z 3 z 4 z 5 z

Well-Being
1 2 3 4 5

Steps   Floors

▷ SUNDAY

BREAKFAST *& Morning* | *Calories* ☕ | **LUNCH** *& Afternoon* | *Calories* ☕ | **DINNER** *& Evening* | *Calories* ☕

Morning Calorie Totals **A** [   ]

Calorie Goal [   ]

Actual (A) + (B) + (C) [   ]

Afternoon Calorie Totals **B** [   ]

☕ [   ]

[   ]

Healthy Options
🥕 🥕 🥕 🥕

Your Five a Day
🍎 🍎 🍎 🍎

Slept Well
①z ②z ③z ④z ⑤z

Well-Being
①☹ ②☹ ③😐 ④🙂 ⑤😊

Evening Calorie Totals **C** [   ]

Steps	Floors
[ ]	[ ]
[ ]	[ ]

▷ WEEK 7 SUMMARY

	Mon	Tue	Wed	Thur	Fri	Sat	Sun
🔥 *Weekly Calorie Totals*							
☕ *Weekly Beverage (No.of ticks) Totals*							
🥕 *Your Vegetable Weekly Totals*							
🍎 *Your Fruit Weekly Totals*							

Your Steps & Floors

35
30
25
15
10
5

Mon Tue Wed Thur Fri Sat Sun

10k
9k
8k
7k
6k
5k
4k

Mon Tue Wed Thur Fri Sat Sun

▷ MONDAY

BREAKFAST *& Morning* Calories ☕ | **LUNCH** *& Afternoon* Calories ☕ | **DINNER** *& Evening* Calories ☕

Morning Calorie Totals Ⓐ

Calorie Goal

Actual Ⓐ + Ⓑ + Ⓒ

Afternoon Calorie Totals Ⓑ

☕

Healthy Options
🥕 🥕 🥕 🥕

Your Five a Day
🍎 🍎 🍎 🍎

Slept Well
①z ②z ③z ④z ⑤z

Well-Being
①☹ ②☹ ③☹ ④☺ ⑤☺

Evening Calorie Totals Ⓒ

Steps   Floors

▷ TUESDAY

BREAKFAST *& Morning* Calories ☕ | **LUNCH** *& Afternoon* Calories ☕ | **DINNER** *& Evening* Calories ☕

Morning Calorie Totals Ⓐ

Calorie Goal

Actual Ⓐ + Ⓑ + Ⓒ

Afternoon Calorie Totals Ⓑ

☕

Healthy Options
🥕 🥕 🥕 🥕

Your Five a Day
🍎 🍎 🍎 🍎

Slept Well
①z ②z ③z ④z ⑤z

Well-Being
①☹ ②☹ ③☹ ④☺ ⑤☺

Evening Calorie Totals Ⓒ

Steps   Floors

▷ WEDNESDAY

BREAKFAST *& Morning* *Calories* ☕ **LUNCH** *& Afternoon* *Calories* ☕ **DINNER** *& Evening* *Calories* ☕

Morning Calorie Totals Ⓐ

Afternoon Calorie Totals Ⓑ

Evening Calorie Totals Ⓒ

Calorie Goal

☕

Healthy Options
🥕 🥕 🥕 🥕

Slept Well
①z ②z ③z ④z ⑤z

Steps **Floors**

Ⓐ + Ⓑ + Ⓒ

Actual

Your Five a Day
🍎 🍎 🍎 🍎

Well-Being
① ② ③ ④ ⑤

▷ THURSDAY

BREAKFAST *& Morning* *Calories* ☕ **LUNCH** *& Afternoon* *Calories* ☕ **DINNER** *& Evening* *Calories* ☕

Morning Calorie Totals Ⓐ

Afternoon Calorie Totals Ⓑ

Evening Calorie Totals Ⓒ

Calorie Goal

☕

Healthy Options
🥕 🥕 🥕 🥕

Slept Well
①z ②z ③z ④z ⑤z

Steps **Floors**

Ⓐ + Ⓑ + Ⓒ

Actual

Your Five a Day
🍎 🍎 🍎 🍎

Well-Being
① ② ③ ④ ⑤

▷ FRIDAY

BREAKFAST *& Morning* Calories

LUNCH *& Afternoon* Calories

DINNER *& Evening* Calories

Morning Calorie Totals **A**

Calorie Goal

Actual **A** + **B** + **C**

Afternoon Calorie Totals **B**

Healthy Options

Your Five a Day

Slept Well
1 z 2 z 3 z 4 z 5 z

Well-Being
1 2 3 4 5

Evening Calorie Totals **C**

Steps Floors

▷ SATURDAY

BREAKFAST *& Morning* Calories

LUNCH *& Afternoon* Calories

DINNER *& Evening* Calories

Morning Calorie Totals **A**

Calorie Goal

Actual **A** + **B** + **C**

Afternoon Calorie Totals **B**

Healthy Options

Your Five a Day

Slept Well
1 z 2 z 3 z 4 z 5 z

Well-Being
1 2 3 4 5

Evening Calorie Totals **C**

Steps Floors

BREAKFAST *& Morning*   *Calories* ☕   **LUNCH** *& Afternoon*   *Calories* ☕   **DINNER** *& Evening*   *Calories* ☕

Morning Calorie Totals Ⓐ

Afternoon Calorie Totals Ⓑ

Evening Calorie Totals Ⓒ

Calorie Goal

Actual   Ⓐ + Ⓑ + Ⓒ

☕

Healthy Options

Slept Well   ① ② ③ ④ ⑤

Steps   Floors

Your Five a Day

Well-Being   ① ② ③ ④ ⑤

▷ WEEK 8 SUMMARY

	Mon	Tue	Wed	Thur	Fri	Sat	Sun

Weekly Calorie Totals

Weekly Beverage (No.of ticks) Totals

Your Vegetable Weekly Totals

Your Fruit Weekly Totals

Your Steps & Floors

35
30
25
15
10
5

Mon   Tue   Wed   Thur   Fri   Sat   Sun

10k
9k
8k
7k
6k
5k
4k

Mon   Tue   Wed   Thur   Fri   Sat   Sun

▷ MONDAY

BREAKFAST *& Morning* *Calories* ☕   **LUNCH** *& Afternoon* *Calories* ☕   **DINNER** *& Evening* *Calories* ☕

Morning Calorie Totals Ⓐ

Afternoon Calorie Totals Ⓑ

Evening Calorie Totals Ⓒ

Calorie Goal

☕

Healthy Options 🥕🥕🥕🥕

Slept Well ①z ②z ③z ④z ⑤z

Steps   Floors

Actual Ⓐ + Ⓑ + Ⓒ

Your Five a Day 🍎🍎🍎🍎

Well-Being ① ② ③ ④ ⑤

▷ TUESDAY

BREAKFAST *& Morning* *Calories* ☕   **LUNCH** *& Afternoon* *Calories* ☕   **DINNER** *& Evening* *Calories* ☕

Morning Calorie Totals Ⓐ

Afternoon Calorie Totals Ⓑ

Evening Calorie Totals Ⓒ

Calorie Goal

☕

Healthy Options 🥕🥕🥕🥕

Slept Well ①z ②z ③z ④z ⑤z

Steps   Floors

Actual Ⓐ + Ⓑ + Ⓒ

Your Five a Day 🍎🍎🍎🍎

Well-Being ① ② ③ ④ ⑤

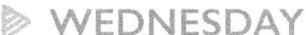 WEDNESDAY

BREAKFAST & *Morning*	*Calories*	LUNCH & *Afternoon*	*Calories*	DINNER & *Evening*	*Calories*

Morning **A**
Calorie Totals

Calorie Goal

Actual Ⓐ + Ⓑ + Ⓒ

Afternoon **B**
Calorie Totals

Evening **C**
Calorie Totals

Healthy Options

Slept Well
①Z ②Z ③Z ④Z ⑤Z

Steps   Floors

Your Five a Day

Well-Being
①☹ ②☹ ③☹ ④☺ ⑤☺

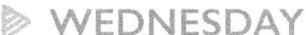 THURSDAY

BREAKFAST & *Morning*	*Calories*	LUNCH & *Afternoon*	*Calories*	DINNER & *Evening*	*Calories*

Morning **A**
Calorie Totals

Calorie Goal

Actual Ⓐ + Ⓑ + Ⓒ

Afternoon **B**
Calorie Totals

Evening **C**
Calorie Totals

Healthy Options

Slept Well
①Z ②Z ③Z ④Z ⑤Z

Steps   Floors

Your Five a Day

Well-Being
①☹ ②☹ ③☹ ④☺ ⑤☺

▷ FRIDAY

BREAKFAST & *Morning* *Calories* ☕ **LUNCH** & *Afternoon* *Calories* ☕ **DINNER** & *Evening* *Calories* ☕

Morning
Calorie Totals (A)

Afternoon
Calorie Totals (B)

Evening
Calorie Totals (C)

Calorie Goal

Actual (A) + (B) + (C)

☕

Healthy Options

Your Five a Day

Slept Well
1 z 2 z 3 z 4 z 5 z

Well-Being
1 2 3 4 5

Steps   Floors

▷ SATURDAY

BREAKFAST & *Morning* *Calories* ☕ **LUNCH** & *Afternoon* *Calories* ☕ **DINNER** & *Evening* *Calories* ☕

Morning
Calorie Totals (A)

Afternoon
Calorie Totals (B)

Evening
Calorie Totals (C)

Calorie Goal

Actual (A) + (B) + (C)

☕

Healthy Options

Your Five a Day

Slept Well
1 z 2 z 3 z 4 z 5 z

Well-Being
1 2 3 4 5

Steps   Floors

⊳ SUNDAY

BREAKFAST *& Morning*   *Calories* ☕   **LUNCH** *& Afternoon*   *Calories* ☕   **DINNER** *& Evening*   *Calories* ☕

Morning Calorie Totals (A)		Afternoon Calorie Totals (B)		Evening Calorie Totals (C)	

Calorie Goal

Actual   (A) + (B) + (C)

Healthy Options

Your Five a Day

Slept Well   1 2 3 4 5

Well-Being   1 2 3 4 5

Steps   Floors

⊳ WEEK 9 SUMMARY

	Mon	Tue	Wed	Thur	Fri	Sat	Sun

Weekly Calorie Totals

Weekly Beverage (No. of ticks) Totals

Your Vegetable Weekly Totals

Your Fruit Weekly Totals

Your Steps & Floors

35
30
25
15
10
5

Mon Tue Wed Thur Fri Sat Sun

10k
9k
8k
7k
6k
5k
4k

Mon Tue Wed Thur Fri Sat Sun

▷ MONDAY

BREAKFAST *& Morning* *Calories* ☕

LUNCH *& Afternoon* *Calories* ☕

DINNER *& Evening* *Calories* ☕

Morning Calorie Totals (A)

Afternoon Calorie Totals (B)

Evening Calorie Totals (C)

Calorie Goal

Actual   (A) + (B) + (C)

☕

Healthy Options

Your Five a Day

Slept Well
1 2 3 4 5

Well-Being
1 2 3 4 5

Steps   Floors

▷ TUESDAY

BREAKFAST *& Morning* *Calories* ☕

LUNCH *& Afternoon* *Calories* ☕

DINNER *& Evening* *Calories* ☕

Morning Calorie Totals (A)

Afternoon Calorie Totals (B)

Evening Calorie Totals (C)

Calorie Goal

Actual   (A) + (B) + (C)

☕

Healthy Options

Your Five a Day

Slept Well
1 2 3 4 5

Well-Being
1 2 3 4 5

Steps   Floors

▷ WEDNESDAY

BREAKFAST *& Morning* Calories ☕   **LUNCH** *& Afternoon* Calories ☕   **DINNER** *& Evening* Calories ☕

Morning Calorie Totals (A)   *Afternoon Calorie Totals* (B)   *Evening Calorie Totals* (C)

Calorie Goal

Actual (A) + (B) + (C)

Healthy Options

Your Five a Day

Slept Well
1 z 2 z 3 z 4 z 5 z

Well-Being
1 2 3 4 5

Steps   Floors

▷ THURSDAY

BREAKFAST *& Morning* Calories ☕   **LUNCH** *& Afternoon* Calories ☕   **DINNER** *& Evening* Calories ☕

Morning Calorie Totals (A)   *Afternoon Calorie Totals* (B)   *Evening Calorie Totals* (C)

Calorie Goal

Actual (A) + (B) + (C)

Healthy Options

Your Five a Day

Slept Well
1 z 2 z 3 z 4 z 5 z

Well-Being
1 2 3 4 5

Steps   Floors

▷ FRIDAY

BREAKFAST *& Morning* *Calories* ☕ | **LUNCH** *& Afternoon* *Calories* ☕ | **DINNER** *& Evening* *Calories* ☕

Morning
Calorie Totals (A) [   ]

Calorie Goal [   ]

Actual (A) + (B) + (C) [   ]

Afternoon
Calorie Totals (B) [   ]

☕ [   ]

[   ]

Healthy Options

Your Five a Day

Evening
Calorie Totals (C) [   ]

Slept Well
1 z 2 z 3 z 4 z 5 z

Well-Being
1 2 3 4 5

Steps **Floors**
[   ] [   ]
[   ] [   ]

▷ SATURDAY

BREAKFAST *& Morning* *Calories* ☕ | **LUNCH** *& Afternoon* *Calories* ☕ | **DINNER** *& Evening* *Calories* ☕

Morning
Calorie Totals (A) [   ]

Calorie Goal [   ]

Actual (A) + (B) + (C) [   ]

Afternoon
Calorie Totals (B) [   ]

☕ [   ]

[   ]

Healthy Options

Your Five a Day

Evening
Calorie Totals (C) [   ]

Slept Well
1 z 2 z 3 z 4 z 5 z

Well-Being
1 2 3 4 5

Steps **Floors**
[   ] [   ]
[   ] [   ]

BREAKFAST *& Morning*   *Calories*   **LUNCH** *& Afternoon*   *Calories*   **DINNER** *& Evening*   *Calories*

Morning
Calorie Totals   (A)

Afternoon
Calorie Totals   (B)

Evening
Calorie Totals   (C)

Calorie Goal

Actual   (A) + (B) + (C)

Healthy Options

Your Five a Day

Slept Well

Well-Being

Steps   Floors

▷ WEEK 10 SUMMARY

	Mon	Tue	Wed	Thur	Fri	Sat	Sun

Weekly Calorie Totals

Weekly Beverage (No.of ticks) Totals

Your Vegetable Weekly Totals

Your Fruit Weekly Totals

Your Steps & Floors

35
30
25
15
10
5

Mon Tue Wed Thur Fri Sat Sun

10k
9k
8k
7k
6k
5k
4k

Mon Tue Wed Thur Fri Sat Sun

▷ MONDAY

BREAKFAST *& Morning* *Calories*   **LUNCH** *& Afternoon* *Calories*   **DINNER** *& Evening* *Calories*

| Morning Calorie Totals **A** | Afternoon Calorie Totals **B** | Evening Calorie Totals **C** |

Calorie Goal

Actual **A** + **B** + **C**

Healthy Options

Your Five a Day

Slept Well
1 2 3 4 5

Well-Being
1 2 3 4 5

Steps   Floors

▷ TUESDAY

BREAKFAST *& Morning* *Calories*   **LUNCH** *& Afternoon* *Calories*   **DINNER** *& Evening* *Calories*

| Morning Calorie Totals **A** | Afternoon Calorie Totals **B** | Evening Calorie Totals **C** |

Calorie Goal

Actual **A** + **B** + **C**

Healthy Options

Your Five a Day

Slept Well
1 2 3 4 5

Well-Being
1 2 3 4 5

Steps   Floors

▷ WEDNESDAY

BREAKFAST *& Morning* *Calories* ☕   **LUNCH** *& Afternoon* *Calories* ☕   **DINNER** *& Evening* *Calories* ☕

Morning
Calorie Totals Ⓐ

Afternoon
Calorie Totals Ⓑ

Evening
Calorie Totals Ⓒ

Calorie Goal

☕

Healthy Options

Slept Well

Steps   Floors

Ⓐ + Ⓑ + Ⓒ

Actual

Your Five a Day

Well-Being

▷ THURSDAY

BREAKFAST *& Morning* *Calories* ☕   **LUNCH** *& Afternoon* *Calories* ☕   **DINNER** *& Evening* *Calories* ☕

Morning
Calorie Totals Ⓐ

Afternoon
Calorie Totals Ⓑ

Evening
Calorie Totals Ⓒ

Calorie Goal

☕

Healthy Options

Slept Well

Steps   Floors

Ⓐ + Ⓑ + Ⓒ

Actual

Your Five a Day

Well-Being

▷ FRIDAY

BREAKFAST & *Morning* *Calories* ☕   **LUNCH** & *Afternoon* *Calories* ☕   **DINNER** & *Evening* *Calories* ☕

Morning
Calorie Totals **A**

Calorie Goal

Actual   **A** + **B** + **C**

Afternoon
Calorie Totals **B**

☕

Healthy Options

Your Five a Day

Slept Well
1 z   2 z   3 z   4 z   5 z

Well-Being
1 ☹   2 ☹   3   4   5 ☺

Evening
Calorie Totals **C**

Steps   Floors

▷ SATURDAY

BREAKFAST & *Morning* *Calories* ☕   **LUNCH** & *Afternoon* *Calories* ☕   **DINNER** & *Evening* *Calories* ☕

Morning
Calorie Totals **A**

Calorie Goal

Actual   **A** + **B** + **C**

Afternoon
Calorie Totals **B**

☕

Healthy Options

Your Five a Day

Slept Well
1 z   2   3 z   4 z   5 z

Well-Being
1 ☹   2 ☹   3   4 ☺   5 ☺

Evening
Calorie Totals **C**

Steps   Floors

BREAKFAST *& Morning* *Calories* ☕   **LUNCH** *& Afternoon* *Calories* ☕   **DINNER** *& Evening* *Calories* ☕

Morning
Calorie Totals Ⓐ

Afternoon
Calorie Totals Ⓑ

Evening
Calorie Totals Ⓒ

Calorie Goal

☕

Healthy Options

Slept Well
① ② ③ ④ ⑤

Steps   Floors

Actual
Ⓐ + Ⓑ + Ⓒ

Your Five a Day

Well-Being
① ② ③ ④ ⑤

▷ WEEK 11 SUMMARY

	Mon	Tue	Wed	Thur	Fri	Sat	Sun

Weekly Calorie Totals

Weekly Beverage (No.of ticks) Totals

Your Vegetable Weekly Totals

Your Fruit Weekly Totals

Your Steps & Floors

35
30
25
15
10
5

Mon Tue Wed Thur Fri Sat Sun

10k
9k
8k
7k
6k
5k
4k

Mon Tue Wed Thur Fri Sat Sun

▷ MONDAY

BREAKFAST *& Morning*   *Calories* ☕   **LUNCH** *& Afternoon*   *Calories* ☕   **DINNER** *& Evening*   *Calories* ☕

Morning Calorie Totals **A** _____   *Afternoon Calorie Totals* **B** _____   *Evening Calorie Totals* **C** _____

Calorie Goal _____   ☕ _____   Healthy Options 🥕🥕🥕🥕   Slept Well ①②③④⑤   Steps   Floors

Actual   **A** + **B** + **C**   _____   Your Five a Day 🍎🍎🍎🍎   Well-Being ①②③④⑤

▷ TUESDAY

BREAKFAST *& Morning*   *Calories* ☕   **LUNCH** *& Afternoon*   *Calories* ☕   **DINNER** *& Evening*   *Calories* ☕

Morning Calorie Totals **A** _____   *Afternoon Calorie Totals* **B** _____   *Evening Calorie Totals* **C** _____

Calorie Goal _____   ☕ _____   Healthy Options 🥕🥕🥕🥕   Slept Well ①②③④⑤   Steps   Floors

Actual   **A** + **B** + **C**   _____   Your Five a Day 🍎🍎🍎🍎   Well-Being ①②③④⑤

WEDNESDAY

BREAKFAST & *Morning*   *Calories*   **LUNCH** & *Afternoon*   *Calories*   **DINNER** & *Evening*   *Calories*

Morning Calorie Totals (A)

Afternoon Calorie Totals (B)

Evening Calorie Totals (C)

Calorie Goal

Healthy Options

Slept Well
1 z 2 z 3 z 4 z 5 z

Steps   Floors

Actual   (A) + (B) + (C)

Your Five a Day

Well-Being
1 2 3 4 5

THURSDAY

BREAKFAST & *Morning*   *Calories*   **LUNCH** & *Afternoon*   *Calories*   **DINNER** & *Evening*   *Calories*

Morning Calorie Totals (A)

Afternoon Calorie Totals (B)

Evening Calorie Totals (C)

Calorie Goal

Healthy Options

Slept Well
1 z 2 z 3 z 4 z 5 z

Steps   Floors

Actual   (A) + (B) + (C)

Your Five a Day

Well-Being
1 2 3 4 5

▷ FRIDAY

BREAKFAST & *Morning* *Calories* ☕   **LUNCH** & *Afternoon* *Calories* ☕   **DINNER** & *Evening* *Calories* ☕

Morning Calorie Totals Ⓐ _____

Afternoon Calorie Totals Ⓑ _____

Evening Calorie Totals Ⓒ _____

Calorie Goal _____

☕ _____

Healthy Options

Slept Well
① ② ③ ④ ⑤
z z z z z

Steps   **Floors**

Actual Ⓐ + Ⓑ + Ⓒ _____

_____

Your Five a Day

Well-Being
① ② ③ ④ ⑤

▷ SATURDAY

BREAKFAST & *Morning* *Calories* ☕   **LUNCH** & *Afternoon* *Calories* ☕   **DINNER** & *Evening* *Calories* ☕

Morning Calorie Totals Ⓐ _____

Afternoon Calorie Totals Ⓑ _____

Evening Calorie Totals Ⓒ _____

Calorie Goal _____

☕ _____

Healthy Options

Slept Well
① ② ③ ④ ⑤
z z z z z

Steps   **Floors**

Actual Ⓐ + Ⓑ + Ⓒ _____

_____

Your Five a Day

Well-Being
① ② ③ ④ ⑤

▷ SUNDAY

BREAKFAST *& Morning*   *Calories* ☕   **LUNCH** *& Afternoon*   *Calories* ☕   **DINNER** *& Evening*   *Calories* ☕

Morning
Calorie Totals **(A)**

Afternoon
Calorie Totals **(B)**

Evening
Calorie Totals **(C)**

Calorie Goal

☕

Actual   (A) + (B) + (C)

Healthy Options

Your Five a Day

Slept Well
(1)z (2)z (3)z (4)z (5)z

Well-Being
(1) (2) (3) (4) (5)

Steps   Floors

▷ WEEK 12 SUMMARY

	Mon	Tue	Wed	Thur	Fri	Sat	Sun

Weekly Calorie Totals

Weekly Beverage (No. of ticks) Totals

Your Vegetable Weekly Totals

Your Fruit Weekly Totals

Your Steps & Floors

35
30
25
15
10
5

Mon Tue Wed Thur Fri Sat Sun

10k
9k
8k
7k
6k
5k
4k

Mon Tue Wed Thur Fri Sat Sun

▷ MONDAY

BREAKFAST *& Morning* *Calories*   **LUNCH** *& Afternoon* *Calories*   **DINNER** *& Evening* *Calories*

Morning Calorie Totals (A)	*Afternoon Calorie Totals* (B)	*Evening Calorie Totals* (C)

Calorie Goal

Actual   (A) + (B) + (C)

Healthy Options

Your Five a Day

Slept Well   1 2 3 4 5

Well-Being   1 2 3 4 5

Steps   Floors

▷ TUESDAY

BREAKFAST *& Morning* *Calories*   **LUNCH** *& Afternoon* *Calories*   **DINNER** *& Evening* *Calories*

Morning Calorie Totals (A)	*Afternoon Calorie Totals* (B)	*Evening Calorie Totals* (C)

Calorie Goal

Actual   (A) + (B) + (C)

Healthy Options

Your Five a Day

Slept Well   1 2 3 4 5

Well-Being   1 2 3 4 5

Steps   Floors

▷ WEDNESDAY

BREAKFAST *& Morning* — Calories ☕   **LUNCH** *& Afternoon* — Calories ☕   **DINNER** *& Evening* — Calories ☕

Morning Calorie Totals (A)

Afternoon Calorie Totals (B)

Evening Calorie Totals (C)

Calorie Goal

Actual (A) + (B) + (C)

Healthy Options

Your Five a Day

Slept Well
1z 2z 3z 4z 5z

Well-Being
1 2 3 4 5

Steps   Floors

▷ THURSDAY

BREAKFAST *& Morning* — Calories ☕   **LUNCH** *& Afternoon* — Calories ☕   **DINNER** *& Evening* — Calories ☕

Morning Calorie Totals (A)

Afternoon Calorie Totals (B)

Evening Calorie Totals (C)

Calorie Goal

Actual (A) + (B) + (C)

Healthy Options

Your Five a Day

Slept Well
1z 2z 3z 4z 5z

Well-Being
1 2 3 4 5

Steps   Floors

▷ FRIDAY

BREAKFAST & *Morning*   *Calories* ☕   **LUNCH** & *Afternoon*   *Calories* ☕   **DINNER** & *Evening*   *Calories* ☕

Morning Calorie Totals (A)   *Afternoon Calorie Totals* (B)   *Evening Calorie Totals* (C)

Calorie Goal   ☕ [ ]   Healthy Options   Slept Well   Steps   Floors

Actual   (A) + (B) + (C)   [ ]   Your Five a Day   Well-Being

▷ SATURDAY

BREAKFAST & *Morning*   *Calories* ☕   **LUNCH** & *Afternoon*   *Calories* ☕   **DINNER** & *Evening*   *Calories* ☕

Morning Calorie Totals (A)   *Afternoon Calorie Totals* (B)   *Evening Calorie Totals* (C)

Calorie Goal   ☕ [ ]   Healthy Options   Slept Well   Steps   Floors

Actual   (A) + (B) + (C)   [ ]   Your Five a Day   Well-Being

▷ SUNDAY

BREAKFAST *& Morning* | *Calories* | ☕ | **LUNCH** *& Afternoon* | *Calories* | ☕ | **DINNER** *& Evening* | *Calories* | ☕

Morning
Calorie Totals Ⓐ

Calorie Goal

Actual Ⓐ + Ⓑ + Ⓒ

Afternoon
Calorie Totals Ⓑ

☕

Evening
Calorie Totals Ⓒ

Healthy Options

Your Five a Day

Slept Well
① ② ③ ④ ⑤

Well-Being
① ② ③ ④ ⑤

Steps **Floors**

▷ WEEK 13 SUMMARY

	Mon	Tue	Wed	Thur	Fri	Sat	Sun

Weekly Calorie Totals

☕ *Weekly Beverage (No.of ticks) Totals*

🥕 *Your Vegetable Weekly Totals*

🍎 *Your Fruit Weekly Totals*

Your Steps & Floors

35
30
25
15
10
5

Mon Tue Wed Thur Fri Sat Sun

10k
9k
8k
7k
6k
5k
4k

Mon Tue Wed Thur Fri Sat Sun

SECTION 3

A Personal Journey About You and Your Body…

It's time to learn what your body can do!

The Body Plan Exercise Programme:

▷ 3 IN A ROW Routine

▷ The Exercises

▷ Workout Log Sheets

▷ Progress Page

LETS GO!

If you are looking to Shape up, Tone or Build Muscle.
Visit our website : www.thebodyplanplus.com Go to Muscle Building !

Amazing Plans Tailored For You - in the Home or in the Gym !

Access Password - **702021**

_____
_____
_____
_____
_____
_____
_____
_____
_____
_____
_____
_____

"The body achieves what the mind believes"

THE "3 IN A ROW" EXERCISE PROGRAMME ▶

We all come in different shapes & sizes and have various levels of stamina, fitness and flexibility. Which is why....The Body Plan Plus Exercise programme has been created to cater for all body types.

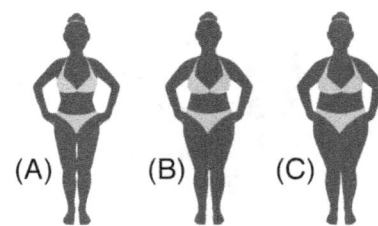

This Exercise Plan is really clever and has been designed to allow you to jump in and get started at your level. You pick the Exercises that are right for your body type and current level of fitness.

(A)   (B)   (C)

Increase your fitness levels at the pace your body will thank you for.
Burn those calories every day without burning yourself out and quitting!

I do not know you personally, and do not know your current weight, levels of fitness or flexibility. So if you feel like I have under-estimated your ability in any way I apologise.

This Exercise Programme (3 IN A ROW) is more of a formula than a routine.
I am not going to tell you which exercises to pick, that's up to you with your honest approach, knowing your own body and what you are capable of doing.

The suggested starting point for everyone is **LEVEL ONE**, and again if you feel my suggested starting point is not enough for you, then please accept my apology. But trust me, you will soon be hitting the levels that push you hard!

The next few pages explain my exercise formula for progressive increases.
The first time you read through, it may look a little complicated, but trust me it isn't. Read it through a couple of times and watch the video attached to these pages on our Website or Facebook page.

This formula is easy, and your body will be grateful you're using it!

The exercises are shown on page 142. Molly the model comes in three body types, A, B and C. For illustration purposes, I am using Molly the model Body Type A.

3 IN A ROW ROUTINE ▶

This is a very clever plan and it is has been created to allow your body to do the talking. As mentioned on Reference pages 173, too much too soon is not the way to build exercise into your life. You need to use the right Exercises for your current level of fitness and body type, then slowly over time increase your intensity by performing more challenging and energy demanding Movements.

Your body will slowly get used to these increases in intensity and resistance, and in a short time you will increase your stamina, fitness levels and lose weight quicker. And all of this will happen without you feeling tired or fatigued, thus avoiding the most common "Give up points".

You can't over do it with the programme, because you can only move up to the next level of intensity when you have completed three exercises routines in a row, hence the name: **3 IN A ROW ROUTINE.**

1   2   3

▷ If you **complete** three exercise routines in a row, you INCREASE your intensity by moving **up** a level.

▷ If you **fail** your routine three times in a row, you REDUCE your intensity by moving **down** a level.

FAIL is a strong word, maybe think on it as NOT completing your exercise routine to your satisfaction - We will talk about this on page 132

To keep track of all this moving up a level and down a level, you keep yourself organised with your:

▷ Work Out Log Sheet
▷ Progress Chart Page

On the next page, we will have a look at your Work out Log Sheet and explain your Progress Chart.

WORKOUT LOG SHEET

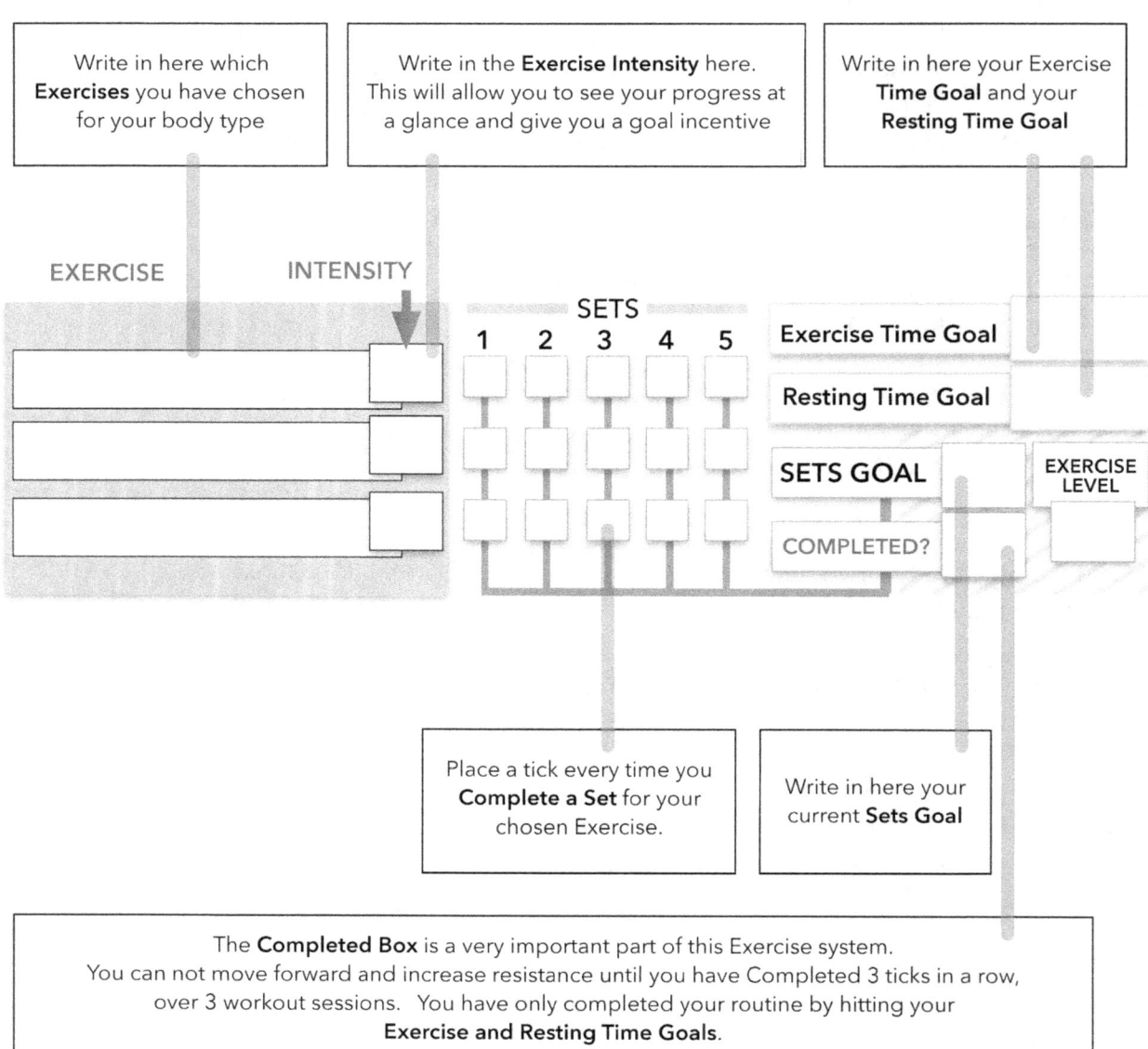

Write in here which **Exercises** you have chosen for your body type

Write in the **Exercise Intensity** here. This will allow you to see your progress at a glance and give you a goal incentive

Write in here your Exercise **Time Goal** and your **Resting Time Goal**

EXERCISE   INTENSITY

SETS

1   2   3   4   5

Exercise Time Goal

Resting Time Goal

SETS GOAL

COMPLETED?

EXERCISE LEVEL

Place a tick every time you **Complete a Set** for your chosen Exercise.

Write in here your current **Sets Goal**

The **Completed Box** is a very important part of this Exercise system. You can not move forward and increase resistance until you have Completed 3 ticks in a row, over 3 workout sessions. You have only completed your routine by hitting your **Exercise and Resting Time Goals**.

EXAMPLE - LEVEL 6

Example: When you are at Level 6 **Your Workout Log Sheet** will look like this.

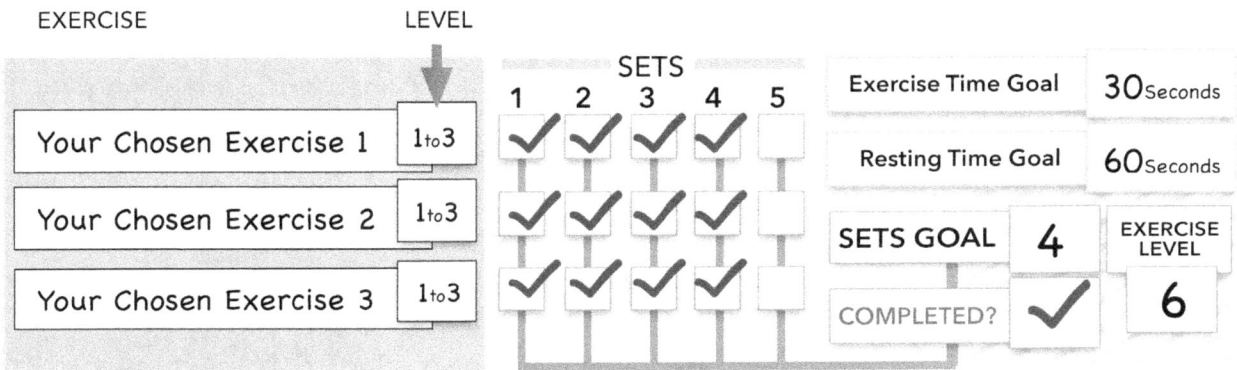

Level 6
3 Exercises
4 Sets For Each Exercise
Exercise Time Goal 30 Seconds
Resting Time Goal **60** Seconds
Total Exercise Workout Time
6 Minutes

ONE LEVEL AT A TIME - FORWARDS & BACKWARDS

Your goal, is for you to keep doing more, without feeling the pain of it all. You have to allow your body time to catch up sometimes, so you have to step back a level. Stepping back is not failure, it's clever and it works. Stepping back a level is simply listening to your body. This is what it needs to do to grow and adapt to it's new physical challenges.

Your exercise routine is all about time. (Exercise Time and Resting Time)

This is how you work it out and when to put a

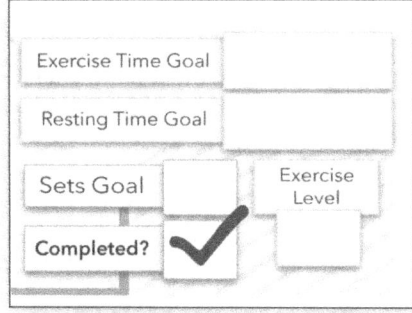

If you complete all your sets for each exercise matching your TIME GOAL and RESTING GOAL then you place a well deserved "TICK" in your **Completed** box.

Then place a **tick** on your Progress Page for the days routine.

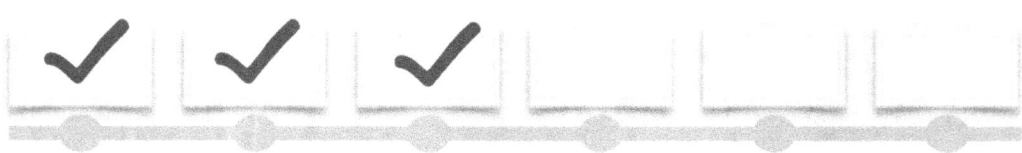

When you have 3 IN ROW, **step up** your intensity and **move up** a level!

Your goal, is for you to keep doing more, but sometimes you just can't hit it. It's really up to you to decide if you have completed your routine by hitting your time goals…. "Did you **end** your exercise a few seconds **before** your goal?" or "Did you **rest** for a little **longer** before starting your next set?" Being honest is going to get you the results you want. If you think you deserve an "X" for the days routine - then give yourself one… Don't feel bad about it, you are listening to your body, and that's going to get you the results you want.

Your exercise routine is all about time. (Exercise Time and Resting Time)

This is how you work it out and when to put a

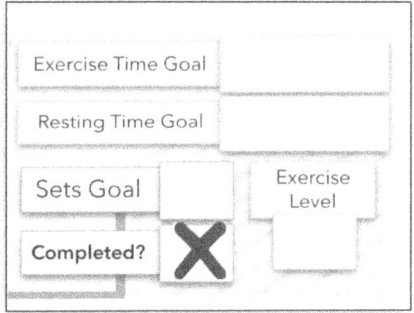

If for any of your Sets, you didn't match your EXERCISE TIME GOAL, or had to rest longer than the RESTING TIME GOAL. Place an "X" in your **Completed** box

Then place a **"X"** on your Progress Page for the days routine.

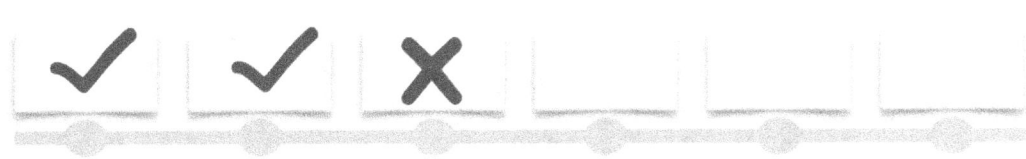

When you have 3 "X's" IN ROW, **step down** your intensity and **move down** a level!

PROGRESS CHART

Pushing yourself does not mean "**Over doing it**". The secret is to allow your body to do the **talking**, listening to it, and **acting** on it. And when you do this the results will be amazing and the process of increasing your fitness levels will be super quick.

The Progress chart on page 169 is your body **talking** to you! And this is how you **act** on the information. (**An Example Progress Page is shown opposite**)

You will Exercise Monday to Saturday (**6 Days Exercising, 1 Day Resting**)

You start at level one on day one. If you complete your routine 3 times in a row you move up to the next level.   Using the example progress page opposite, you can see from (**Exercise Day 1 to Day 27**) the routine has been completed every session.   By now you should be up to level 10 and the intensity starts to increase more and more!

Then as the Levels get harder, you will notice a few "X"s appearing.
(*This is not failure, this is you listening to your body*)

Follow this pattern - It's easy and your body will love you for it!

▶ If you place a tick three times in a row, **INCREASE** your intensity by one level.

▶ If you place an "X" three days in a row **REDUCE** your intensity by one level.

Follow this guide, even if your "**3 IN A ROW**" is broken by a day off for any reason or the resting day which is (Sunday)

As you progress, you will move forward, back, forward, forward and step backwards....

When you progress, you will see a lot more "Moving Forwards" than "Moving Backwards"

And this is the best way to listen to your body, and in doing so, you will not hit those horrible "give up points". **Sustainability is the key to your success.**

You should be able to "Smash" your way through Levels 1 - 5 and this will bring you into the middle of Week 3. Some of you will be able to continue on with plenty of ticks and move through the levels quicker than others. Regardless of the current progress made, fast or slow, the important thing is you did it.

You are training your brain as well as your body, and this "slower approach" has allowed you to concentrate on building up a Routine!   And this means performing a repetitive daily task and building exercise into your life.

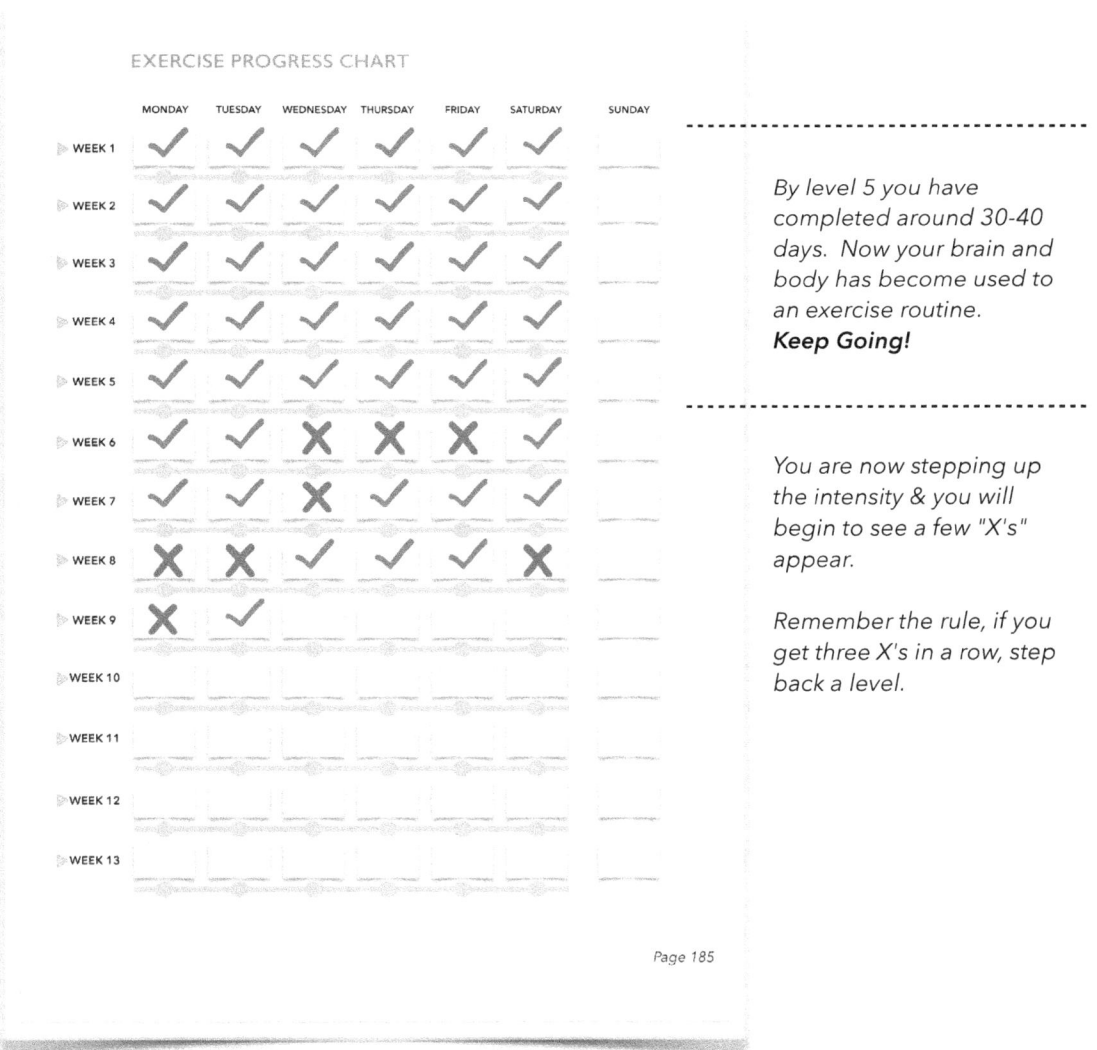

EXERCISE PROGRESS CHART

By level 5 you have completed around 30-40 days. Now your brain and body has become used to an exercise routine. ***Keep Going!***

You are now stepping up the intensity & you will begin to see a few "X's" appear.

Remember the rule, if you get three X's in a row, step back a level.

Page 185

THE EXERCISES

▷ Your Exercises	Intensity	Form Difficulty	Suggested
Box Step	1	1	A,B,C
The Plank	1	2	A,B,C
Leg Raises	2	2	A,B
Chair/Sofa Squat	2	1	A,B,C
Quarter Squat	2	1	B,C
Half Jacks	2	2	A,B,C
Push Ups/Knee	3	3	A,B
Lunges	3	3	A,B
Free Squats	3	3	A,B,C
Stair Walking	3	1	A,B,C
Wall Squats	3	3	A,B
High Knees	4	3	A,B
Jumping Jacks	4	2	A,B
Mountain Climbs	4	4	A
Thrust Squats/Burpees	4	4	A

You will notice that I have built in a guide to Intensity and Difficulty. Use this guide when selecting your exercises...

*For example: Walking up a flight of stairs is relatively easy (**Form Difficulty Rating 1**) But repeat the process for 60 Seconds and it gets quite intensive (**Intensity Rating 3**)*

*The same applies for the other exercises, so choose wisely - **Good Luck!***

Exercise Routine
Levels 1 - 4

▷ Your exercise routine progresses in intensity by altering Exercise and Resting times against Sets performed.

▷ The final increase comes by adding harder more intense Exercises. *But only do this when you have reached level 16 with your First selected Exercises.*

▷ **Level 1**
2 Exercises
2 Sets For Each Exercise
Exercise Time Goal 30 Seconds
Resting Time Goal **60** Seconds
Total Exercise Workout Time
2 Minutes

▷ **Level 2**
2 Exercises
3 Sets For Each Exercise
Exercise Time Goal 30 Seconds
Resting Time Goal **60** Seconds
Total Exercise Workout Time
3 Minutes

▷ **Level 3**
2 Exercises
4 Sets For Each Exercise
Exercise Time Goal 30 Seconds
Resting Time Goal **60** Seconds
Total Exercise Workout Time
4 Minutes

▷ **Level 4**
2 Exercises
5 Sets For Each Exercise
Exercise Time Goal 30 Seconds
Resting Time Goal **60** Seconds
Total Exercise Workout Time
5 Minutes

Exercise Routine Levels 5 - 8

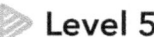 **Level 5**

3 Exercises
3 Sets For Each Exercise
Exercise Time Goal 30 Seconds
Resting Time Goal **60** Seconds
Total Exercise Workout Time
4 Minutes 30 Seconds

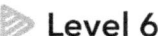 **Level 6**

3 Exercises
4 Sets For Each Exercise
Exercise Time Goal 30 Seconds
Resting Time Goal **60** Seconds
Total Exercise Workout Time
6 Minutes

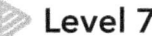 **Level 7**

3 Exercises
5 Sets For Each Exercise
Exercise Time Goal 30 Seconds
Resting Time Goal **60** Seconds
Total Exercise Workout Time
7 Minutes 30 Seconds

Level 8

3 Exercises
2 Sets For Each Exercise
Exercise Time Goal 45 Seconds
Resting Time Goal **60** Seconds
Total Exercise Workout Time
4 Minutes 30 Seconds

Exercise Routine
Levels 9 - 12

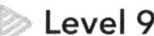 **Level 9**
3 Exercises
3 Sets For Each Exercise
Exercise Time Goal **45** Seconds
Resting Time Goal **60** Seconds
Total Exercise Workout Time
6 Minutes 45 Seconds

Level 10
3 Exercises
4 Sets For Each Exercise
Exercise Time Goal **45** Seconds
Resting Time Goal **60** Seconds
Total Exercise Workout Time
9 Minutes

Level 11
3 Exercises
3 Sets For Each Exercise
Exercise Time Goal **60** Seconds
Resting Time Goal **60** Seconds
Total Exercise Workout Time
9 Minutes

Level 12
3 Exercises
4 Sets For Each Exercise
Exercise Time Goal **60** Seconds
Resting Time Goal **60** Seconds
Total Exercise Workout Time
12 Minutes

Exercise Routine Levels 13 - 16

As the levels get harder the number of sets you perform for each exercise may go up and down, but this is in line with the increased exercise time and reduced resting times.

Level 13
2 Exercises
3 Sets For Each Exercise
Exercise Time Goal **60** Seconds
Resting Time Goal **45** Seconds
Total Exercise Workout Time
6 Minutes

Level 14
2 Exercises
4 Sets For Each Exercise
Exercise Time Goal **60** Seconds
Resting Time Goal **45** Seconds
Total Exercise Workout Time
8 Minutes

Level 15
3 Exercises
2 Sets For Each Exercise
Exercise Time Goal "**60**" Seconds
Resting Time Goal "**30**" Seconds
Total Exercise Workout Time
6 Minutes

Level 16
3 Exercises
3 Sets For Each Exercise
Exercise Time Goal "**60**" Seconds
Resting Time Goal "**30**" Seconds
Total Exercise Workout Time
9 Minutes

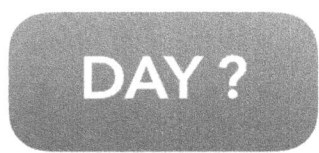

DAY ?

When you reach level 16, performing the maximum intensity exercises your workout log sheet will look like this:

And if you can do this, you have become super, super fit!

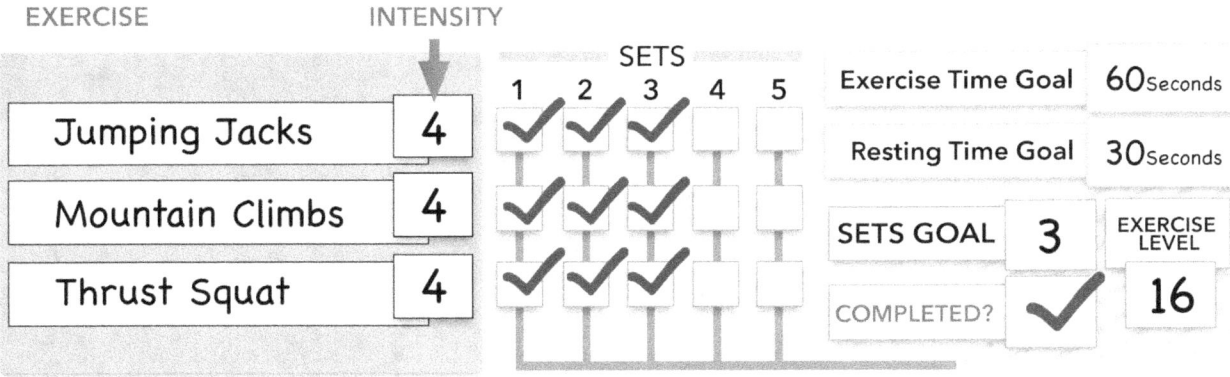

YOUR STARTING POINT

The starting point for everyone is:

Level 1
3 Exercises (*Chosen for your recommended body type*)
2 Sets of each Exercise
30 Seconds for your Exercise Time
60 Seconds for your Resting Time

* You may think this is not enough exercise for you? You may be right, you may be wrong!

If we are wrong it will simply mean you will progress quicker. Don't worry you will soon be up to the correct level of fitness for your body, and then using this formula you will be able to increase your fitness and speed up your weight loss.

Choose one exercise with a level rating of **1** and another exercise with a level rating of **2** or **3**

HIT YOUR TIME GOALS

Exercise and Rest within your 100% Time Goals, *if you can!*

Exercise Time Goal

Exercise for Your Exercise Time Goal Only.
No More, No Less...

Resting Time Goal

Rest only for Your Resting Time Goal Only.
No More, No Less...

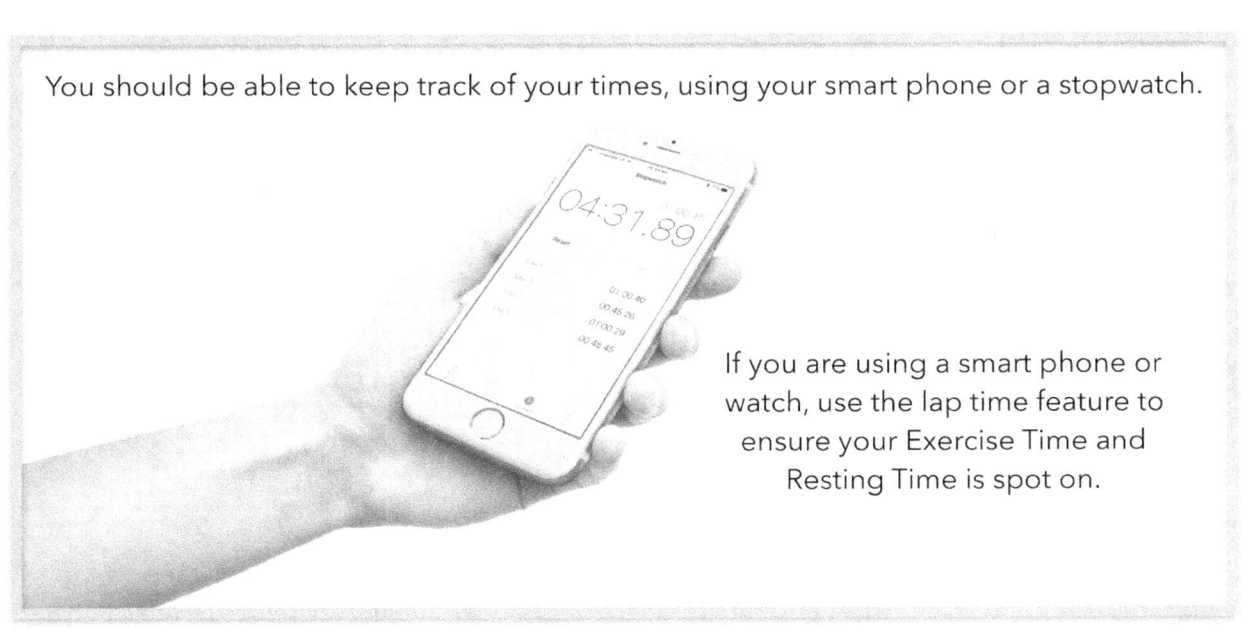

You should be able to keep track of your times, using your smart phone or a stopwatch.

04:31.89

If you are using a smart phone or watch, use the lap time feature to ensure your Exercise Time and Resting Time is spot on.

The Box Step
*Intensity Level **1***
*Difficulty Level **1***

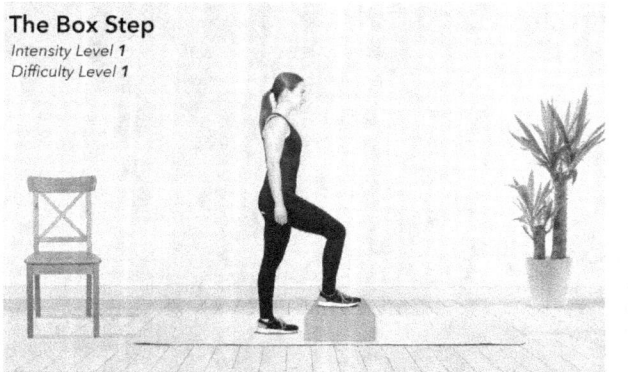

From a standing position take one step on and one step off. Use the bottom step of your stairs. Repeat as fast as possible without losing your balance.

The Plank
*Intensity Level **1***
*Difficulty Level **2***

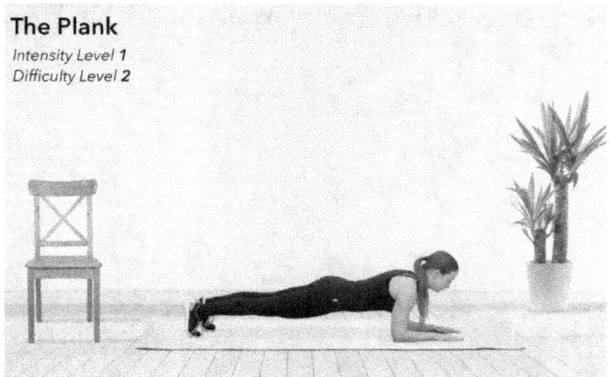

Get into the pushup position on the floor. Now bend your elbows and rest your weight on your forearms. Your elbows should be directly beneath your shoulders, and keeping your body in a straight line without raising your bum. Hold this position for your specified time.

Leg Raises
*Intensity Level **2***
*Difficulty Level **2***

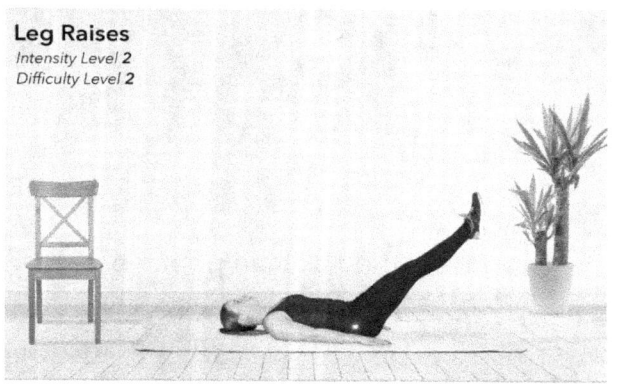

In a lying position, raise your legs about 12 inches from the floor, hold for a few seconds and repeat. Use your arms for balance and to aid the movement. A small beanbag will aid you. If you feel pain in your middle or lower back, stop this exercise until your flexibility and strength has improved.

Chair/Sofa Squat
*Intensity Level **2***
*Difficulty Level **1***

As it say's "On the tin" From a seated position, stand up and then sit down. Perform as fast as possible and swing your arms out to aid in your stand up motion. You can remain seated for 1 to 2 seconds if required.

Quarter Squats

*Intensity Level **2***
*Difficulty Level **1***

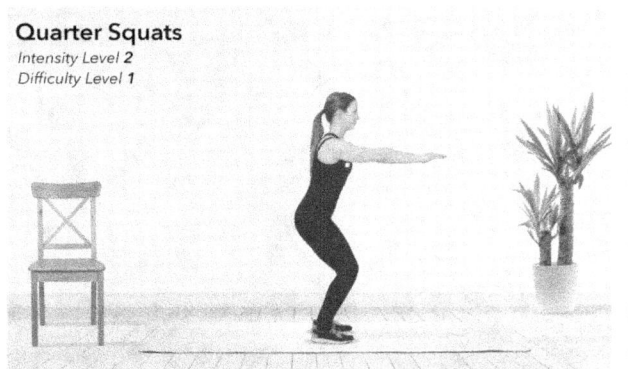

The same as a squat, but instead of lowering yourself so your thighs are parallel to the floor, you only squat to about 45 degrees. You will feel the tension in your thighs and this is what counts. As you get used to this movement you can extend your range until you are performing a full squat.

Half Jacks

*Intensity Level **2***
*Difficulty Level **2***

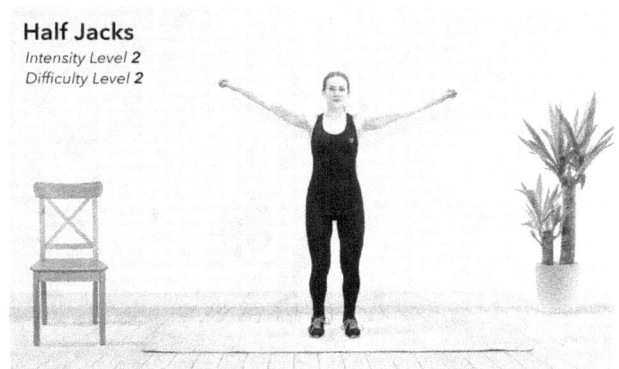

Jumping jacks get your heart pumping. Bend your knees to get the spring, but instead of jumping with your feet wide apart, only jump with them a few inches apart. In time when you get used to the movement you can jump with your feet wider apart. Continue this pattern over time until you are performing a standard jumping jack.

Knee Push Ups

*Intensity Level **3***
*Difficulty Level **3***

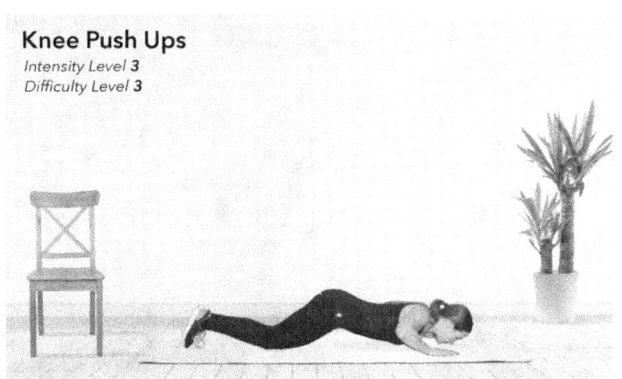

Perform a standard push up or knee push up. The same as regular push ups, but your body weight is on your knees instead of your toes. Lower yourself down until your chest touches the floor and push yourself back up into the starting position.

Lunges

*Intensity Level **3***
*Difficulty Level **3***

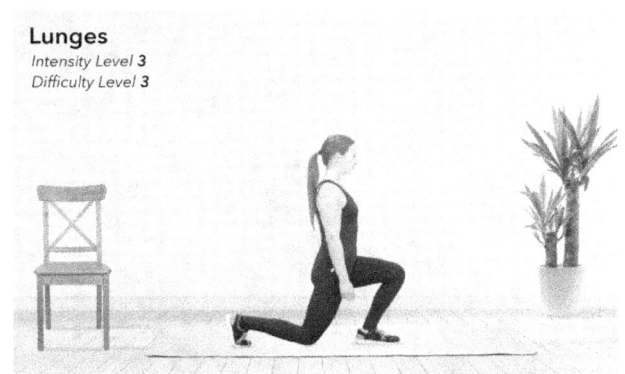

From a standing position, lunge forward on one leg until your thigh is parallel with the floor. Place your hands on your thigh for balance. Thrust yourself back into the starting position and repeat.

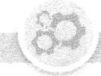

Free Squats
Intensity Level 3
Difficulty Level 3

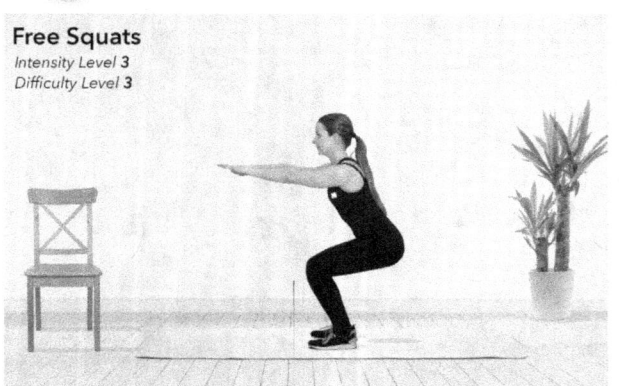

From a standing position, squat down until your thighs are parallel with floor. You can hold this position for a second or two before returning to the starting position.

Stair Walking
Intensity Level 3
Difficulty Level 1

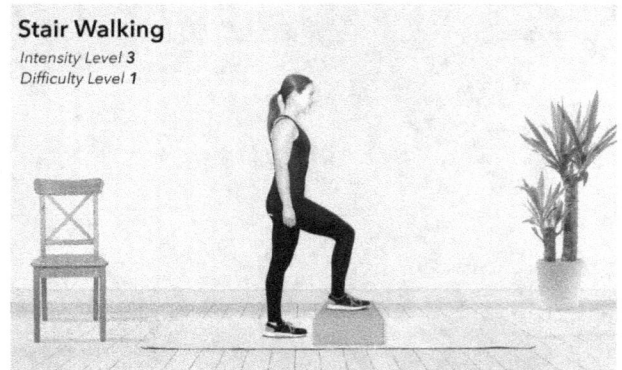

As it say's "On the tin" Try and move at a faster pace than normal. Keep your hand on the hand rail and let the rail run through your hands to keep you safe and steady.

Wall Squat
Intensity Level 3
Difficulty Level 3

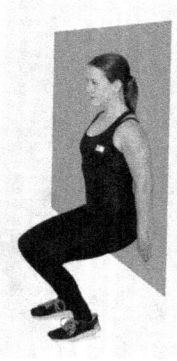

From a standing position, lean against the wall and squat down until your thighs are parallel with the floor. You can hold this position for a second or two before returning to the starting position. This movement is harder than you think, and you may find free squats easier to perform.

High Knees
Intensity Level 4
Difficulty Level 3

Just like jogging on the spot, but raise your knees as high as you can. Perform this exercise as fast as you can without losing your balance. Support yourself with a chair if required.

Jumping Jacks
Intensity Level 4
Difficulty Level 2

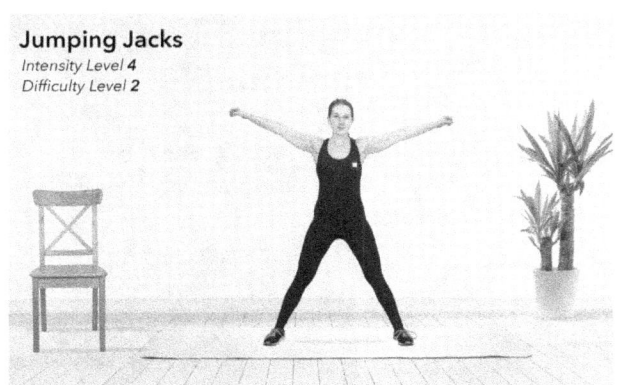

Mountain Climbs
Intensity Level 4
Difficulty Level 4

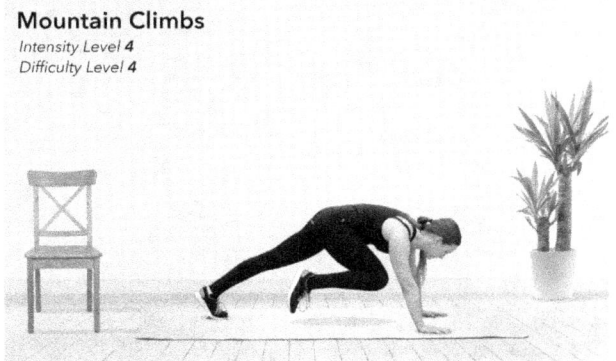

From a standing upright position, jump into a star position with your legs parallel with your shoulders. Clap your hands above your head and then instantly jump back to the starting position.

From the starting PLANK position, thrust your legs alternatively up to your chest in a running motion or "climbing motion" This is a Pro exercise and your body should be ready for it before you try it. You need lots of energy and flexibility for this one.

Thrust Squat Jump/Burpees
Intensity Level 4
Difficulty Level 4

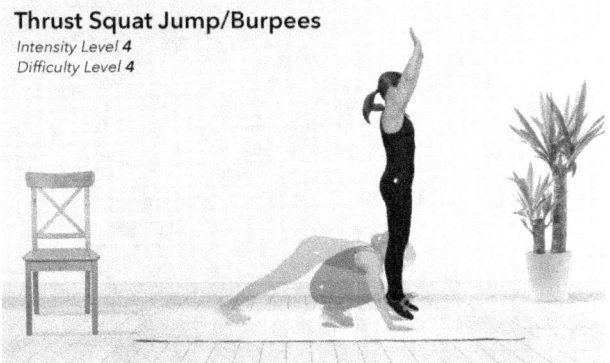

From a standing position, squat down and place your hands on the floor between your knees and thrust your legs back into the plank position. In one continuous movement thrust your legs back into the squat position and then jump up and repeat.

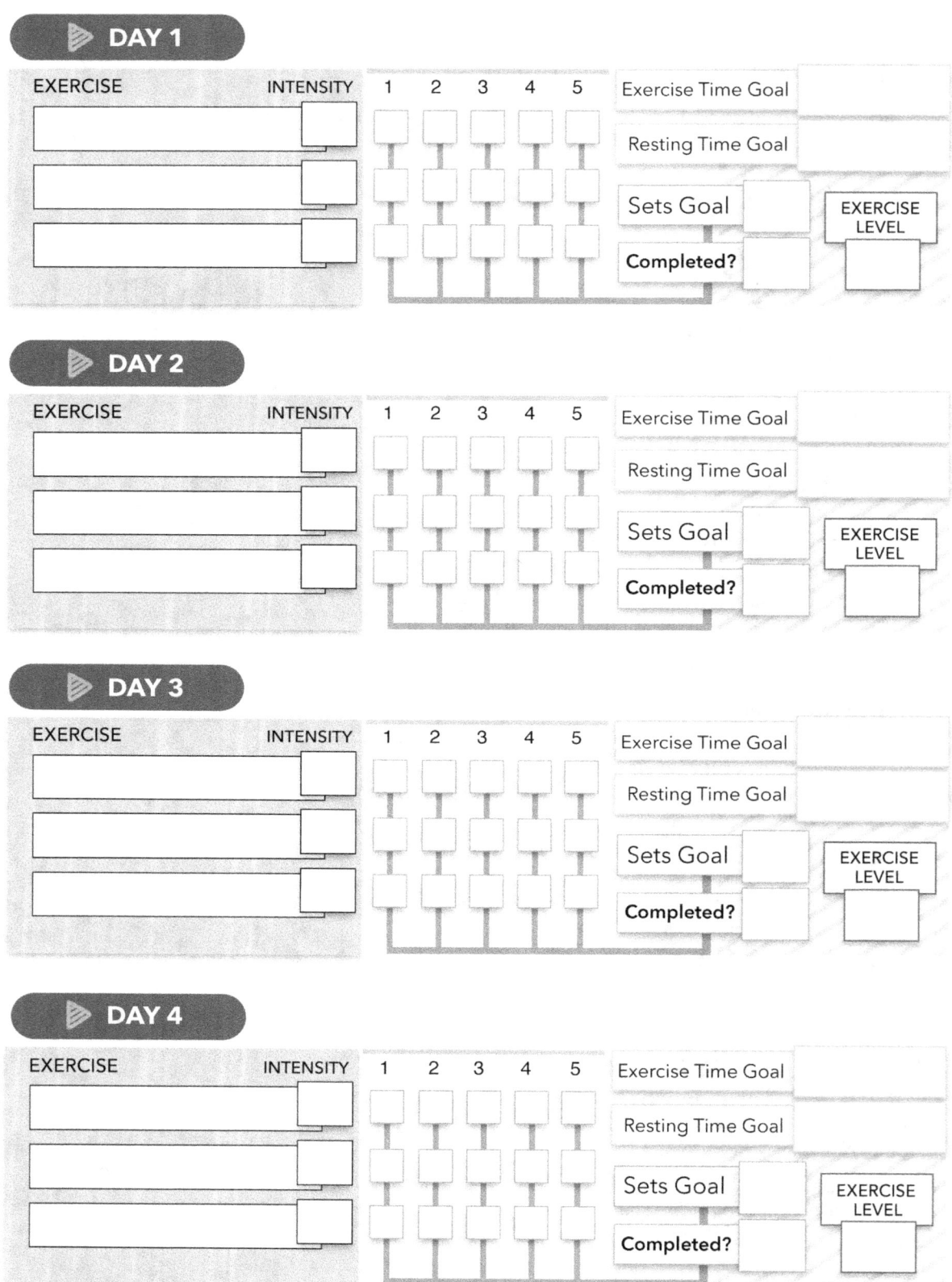

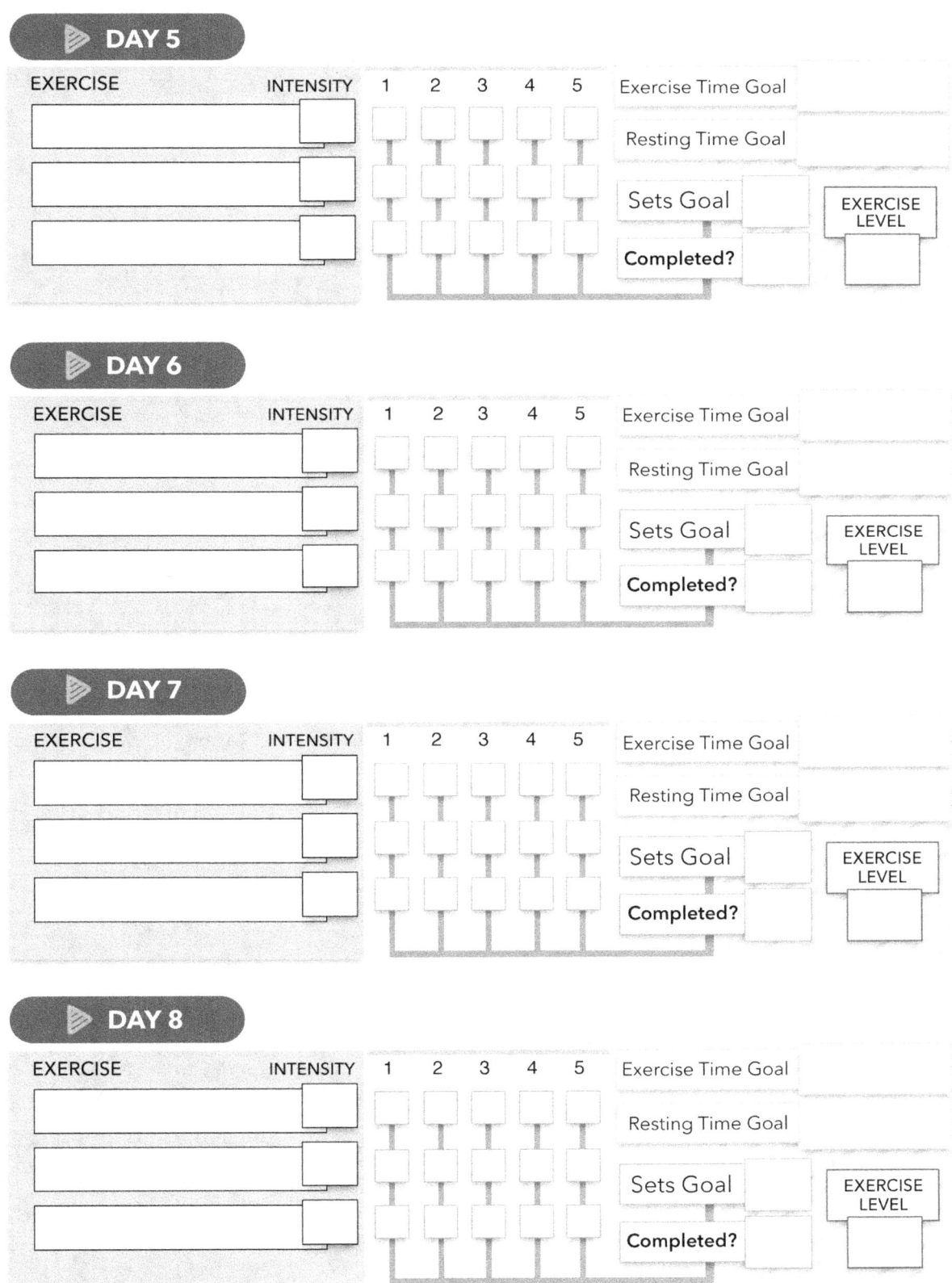

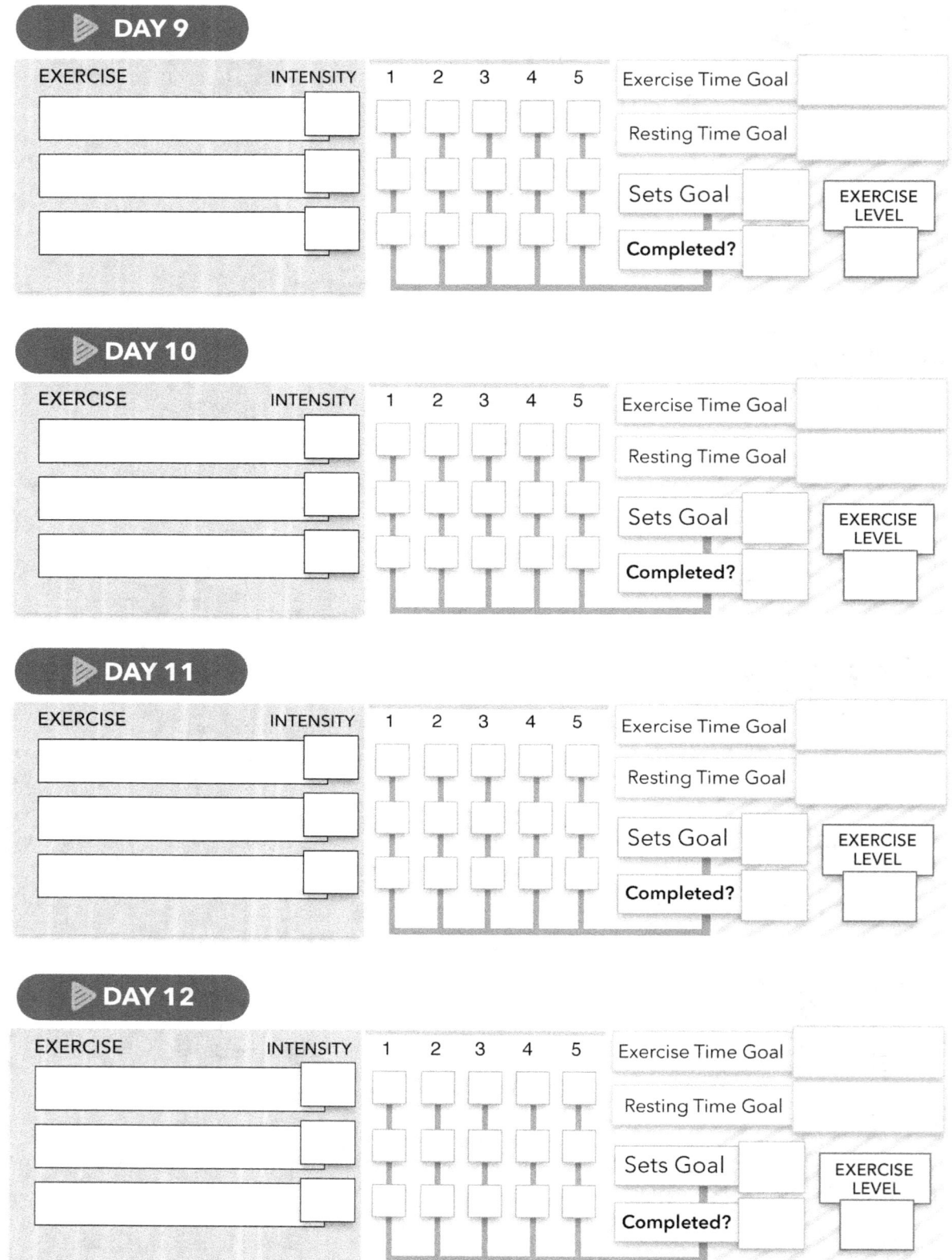

DAY 9

EXERCISE · INTENSITY · 1 2 3 4 5 · Exercise Time Goal · Resting Time Goal · Sets Goal · Completed? · EXERCISE LEVEL

DAY 10

EXERCISE · INTENSITY · 1 2 3 4 5 · Exercise Time Goal · Resting Time Goal · Sets Goal · Completed? · EXERCISE LEVEL

DAY 11

EXERCISE · INTENSITY · 1 2 3 4 5 · Exercise Time Goal · Resting Time Goal · Sets Goal · Completed? · EXERCISE LEVEL

DAY 12

EXERCISE · INTENSITY · 1 2 3 4 5 · Exercise Time Goal · Resting Time Goal · Sets Goal · Completed? · EXERCISE LEVEL

▷ DAY 13

EXERCISE | INTENSITY | 1 2 3 4 5 | Exercise Time Goal
Resting Time Goal
Sets Goal
Completed?
EXERCISE LEVEL

▷ DAY 14

EXERCISE | INTENSITY | 1 2 3 4 5 | Exercise Time Goal
Resting Time Goal
Sets Goal
Completed?
EXERCISE LEVEL

▷ DAY 15

EXERCISE | INTENSITY | 1 2 3 4 5 | Exercise Time Goal
Resting Time Goal
Sets Goal
Completed?
EXERCISE LEVEL

▷ DAY 16

EXERCISE | INTENSITY | 1 2 3 4 5 | Exercise Time Goal
Resting Time Goal
Sets Goal
Completed?
EXERCISE LEVEL

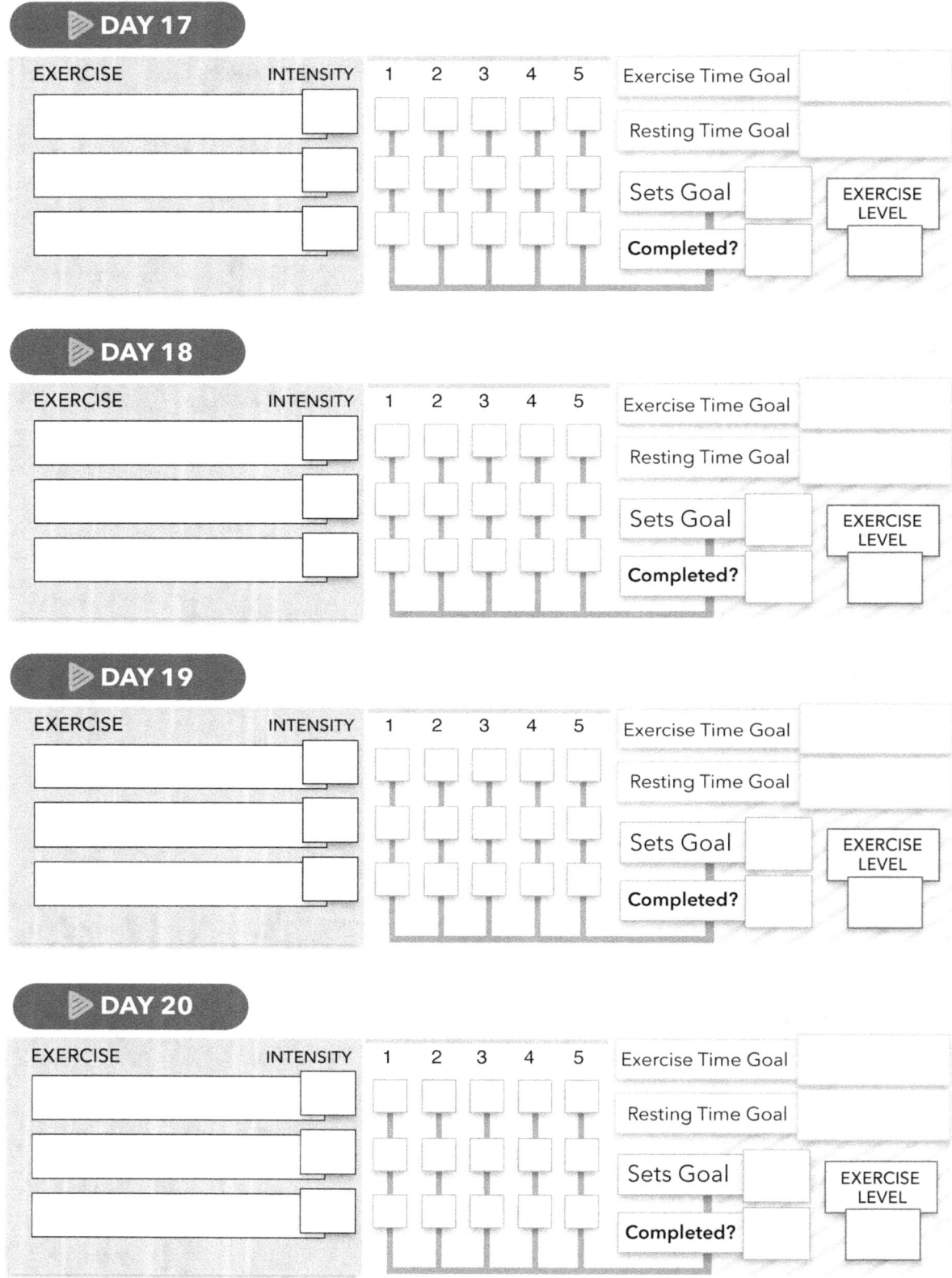

DAY 17

EXERCISE | INTENSITY | 1 2 3 4 5
Exercise Time Goal
Resting Time Goal
Sets Goal
Completed?
EXERCISE LEVEL

DAY 18

EXERCISE | INTENSITY | 1 2 3 4 5
Exercise Time Goal
Resting Time Goal
Sets Goal
Completed?
EXERCISE LEVEL

DAY 19

EXERCISE | INTENSITY | 1 2 3 4 5
Exercise Time Goal
Resting Time Goal
Sets Goal
Completed?
EXERCISE LEVEL

DAY 20

EXERCISE | INTENSITY | 1 2 3 4 5
Exercise Time Goal
Resting Time Goal
Sets Goal
Completed?
EXERCISE LEVEL

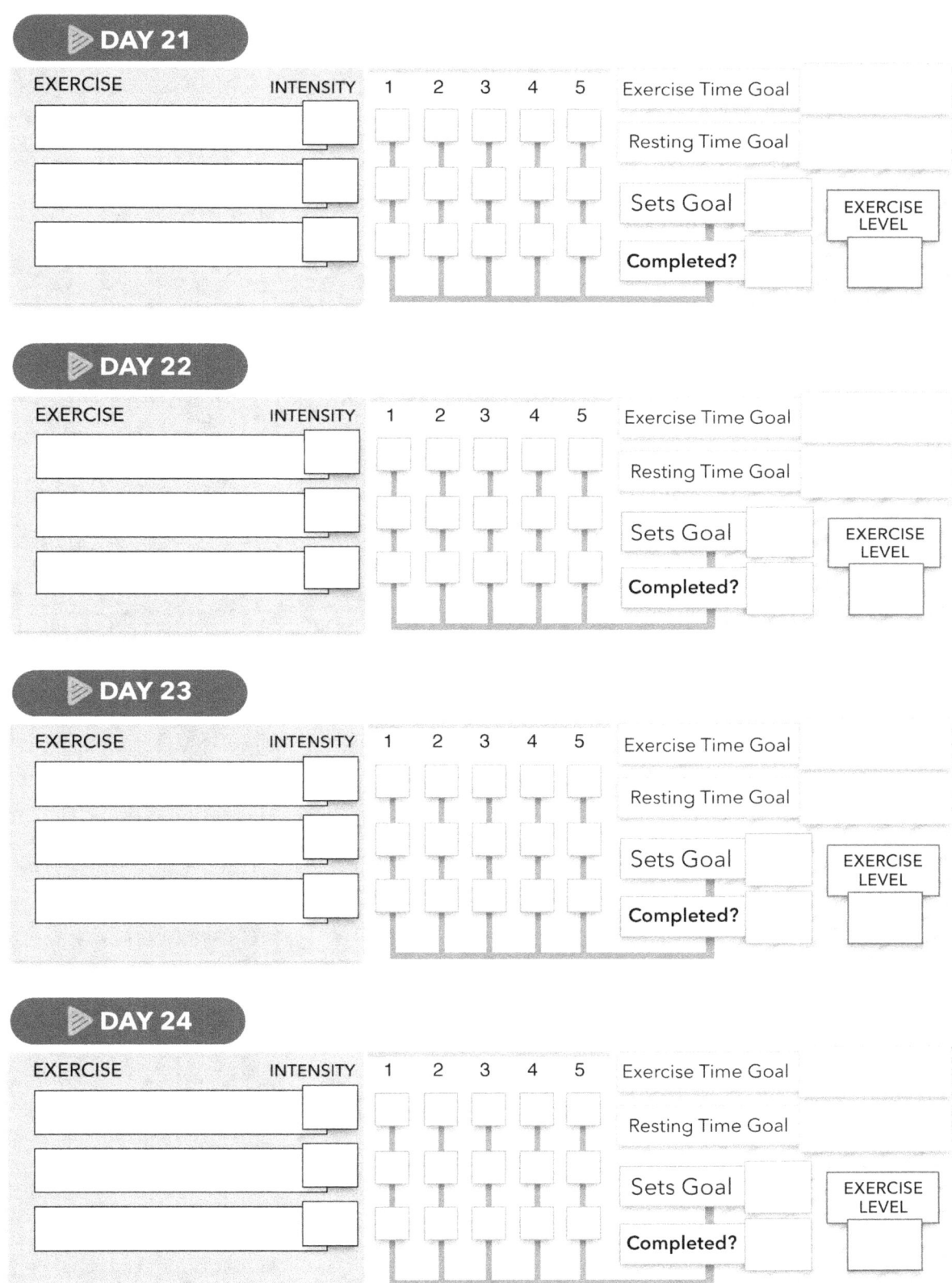

DAY 21

EXERCISE | INTENSITY | 1 2 3 4 5

Exercise Time Goal

Resting Time Goal

Sets Goal

Completed?

EXERCISE LEVEL

DAY 22

EXERCISE | INTENSITY | 1 2 3 4 5

Exercise Time Goal

Resting Time Goal

Sets Goal

Completed?

EXERCISE LEVEL

DAY 23

EXERCISE | INTENSITY | 1 2 3 4 5

Exercise Time Goal

Resting Time Goal

Sets Goal

Completed?

EXERCISE LEVEL

DAY 24

EXERCISE | INTENSITY | 1 2 3 4 5

Exercise Time Goal

Resting Time Goal

Sets Goal

Completed?

EXERCISE LEVEL

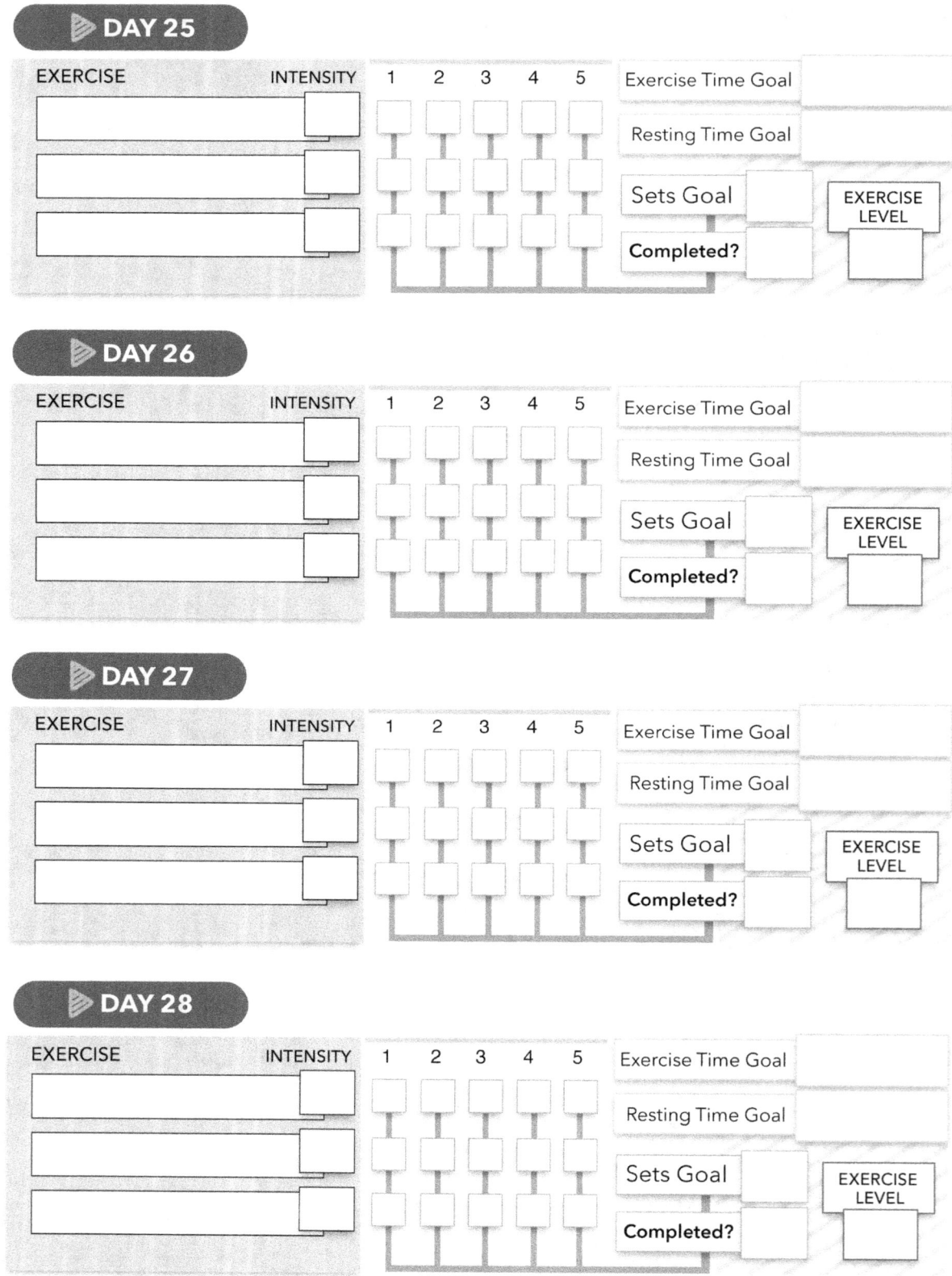

DAY 25

EXERCISE	INTENSITY

1 2 3 4 5

Exercise Time Goal
Resting Time Goal
Sets Goal
Completed?
EXERCISE LEVEL

DAY 26

EXERCISE	INTENSITY

1 2 3 4 5

Exercise Time Goal
Resting Time Goal
Sets Goal
Completed?
EXERCISE LEVEL

DAY 27

EXERCISE	INTENSITY

1 2 3 4 5

Exercise Time Goal
Resting Time Goal
Sets Goal
Completed?
EXERCISE LEVEL

DAY 28

EXERCISE	INTENSITY

1 2 3 4 5

Exercise Time Goal
Resting Time Goal
Sets Goal
Completed?
EXERCISE LEVEL

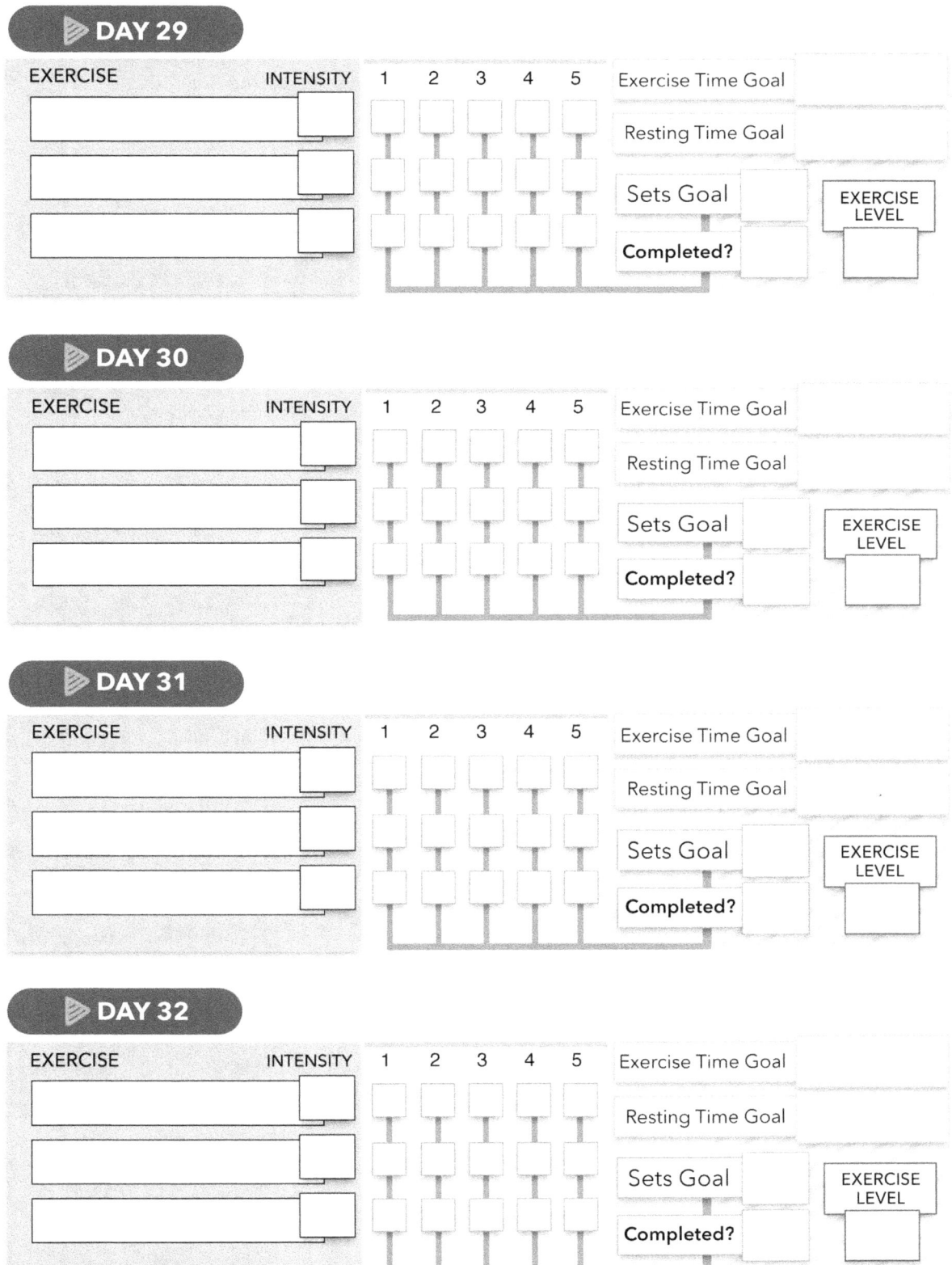

DAY 29

EXERCISE   INTENSITY

1   2   3   4   5

Exercise Time Goal

Resting Time Goal

Sets Goal

Completed?

EXERCISE LEVEL

DAY 30

EXERCISE   INTENSITY

1   2   3   4   5

Exercise Time Goal

Resting Time Goal

Sets Goal

Completed?

EXERCISE LEVEL

DAY 31

EXERCISE   INTENSITY

1   2   3   4   5

Exercise Time Goal

Resting Time Goal

Sets Goal

Completed?

EXERCISE LEVEL

DAY 32

EXERCISE   INTENSITY

1   2   3   4   5

Exercise Time Goal

Resting Time Goal

Sets Goal

Completed?

EXERCISE LEVEL

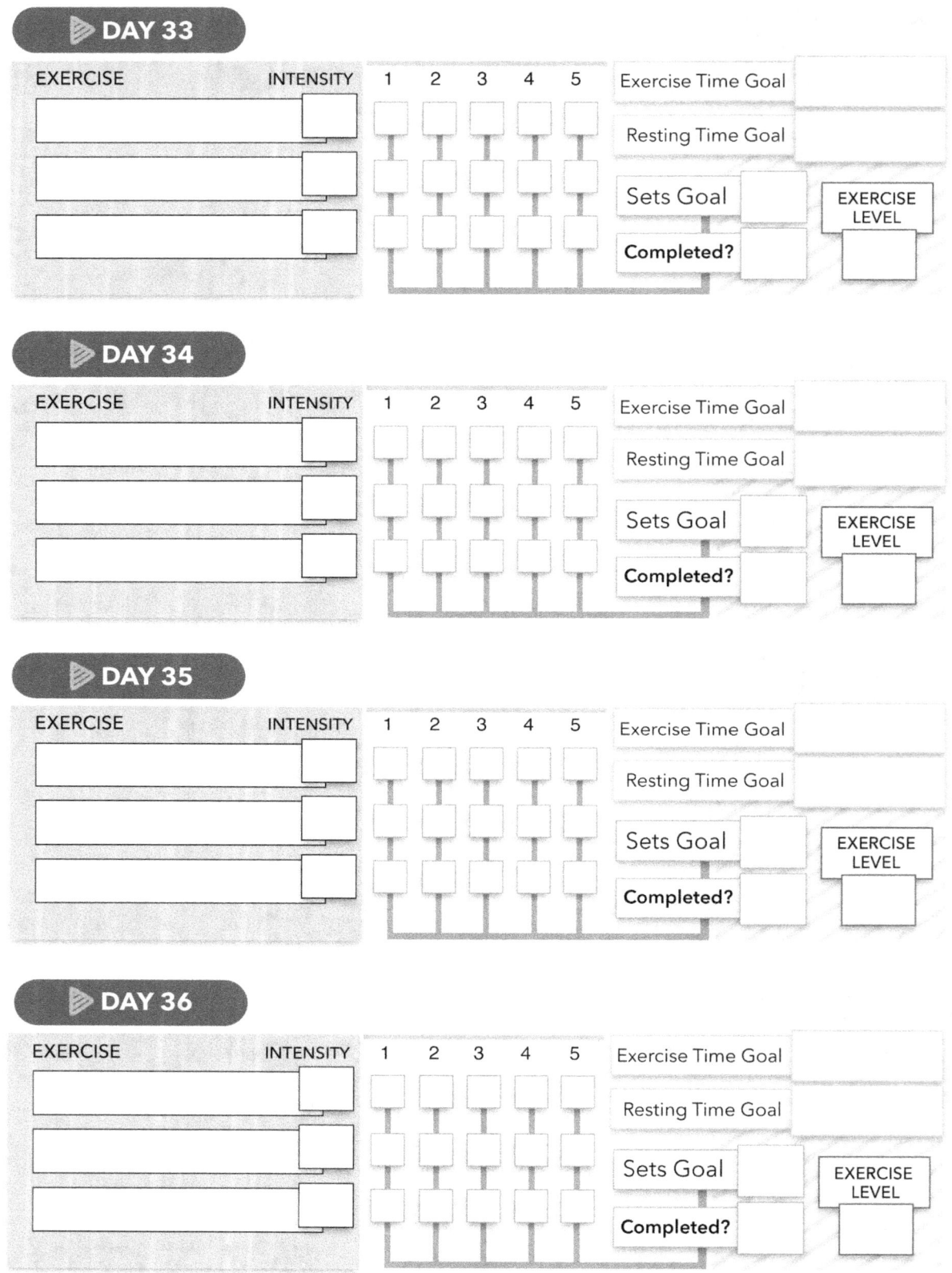

DAY 33

EXERCISE | INTENSITY

1 2 3 4 5

Exercise Time Goal

Resting Time Goal

Sets Goal

Completed?

EXERCISE LEVEL

DAY 34

EXERCISE | INTENSITY

1 2 3 4 5

Exercise Time Goal

Resting Time Goal

Sets Goal

Completed?

EXERCISE LEVEL

DAY 35

EXERCISE | INTENSITY

1 2 3 4 5

Exercise Time Goal

Resting Time Goal

Sets Goal

Completed?

EXERCISE LEVEL

DAY 36

EXERCISE | INTENSITY

1 2 3 4 5

Exercise Time Goal

Resting Time Goal

Sets Goal

Completed?

EXERCISE LEVEL

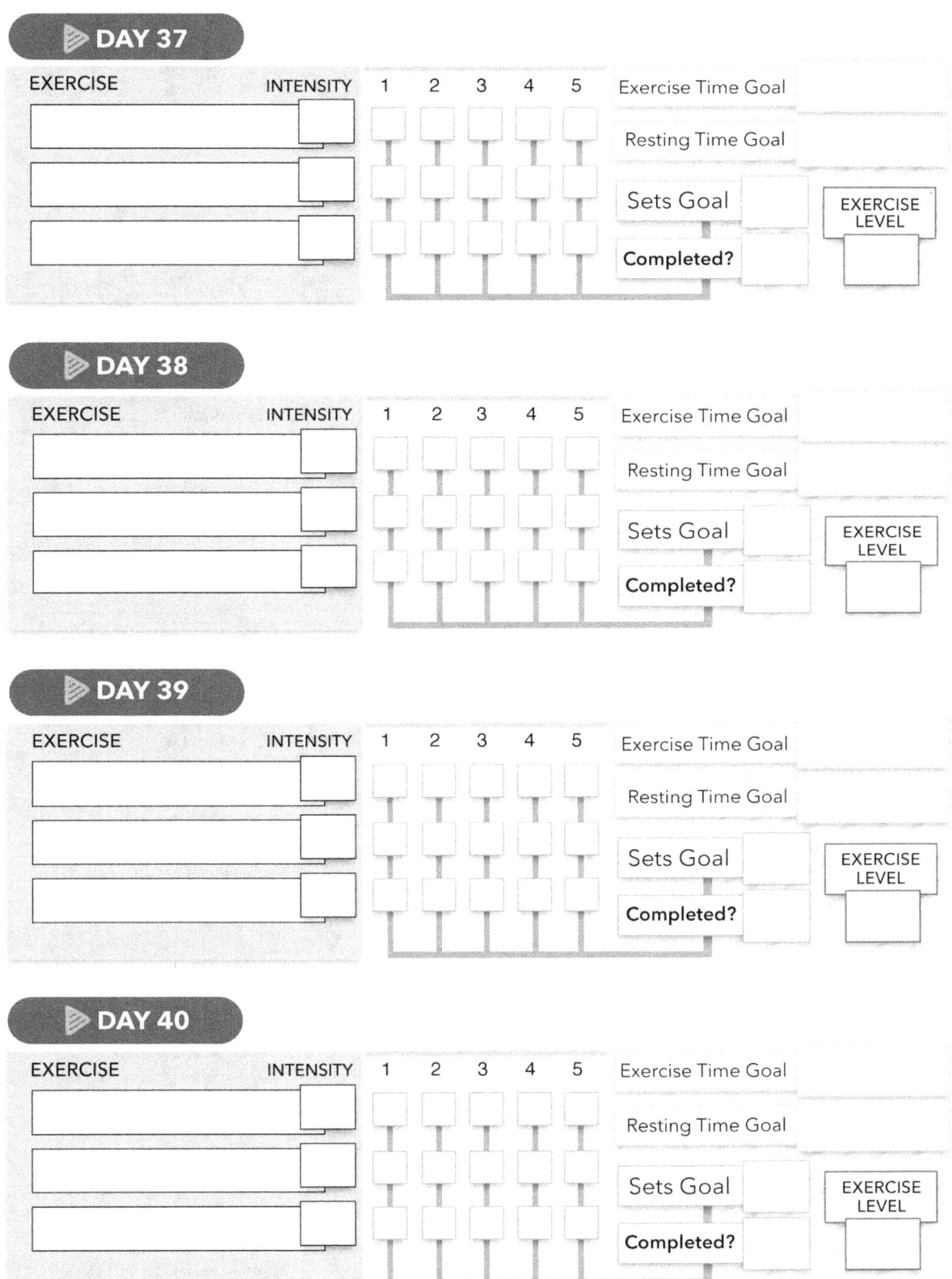

DAY 37

EXERCISE · INTENSITY · 1 2 3 4 5 · Exercise Time Goal · Resting Time Goal · Sets Goal · Completed? · EXERCISE LEVEL

DAY 38

EXERCISE · INTENSITY · 1 2 3 4 5 · Exercise Time Goal · Resting Time Goal · Sets Goal · Completed? · EXERCISE LEVEL

DAY 39

EXERCISE · INTENSITY · 1 2 3 4 5 · Exercise Time Goal · Resting Time Goal · Sets Goal · Completed? · EXERCISE LEVEL

DAY 40

EXERCISE · INTENSITY · 1 2 3 4 5 · Exercise Time Goal · Resting Time Goal · Sets Goal · Completed? · EXERCISE LEVEL

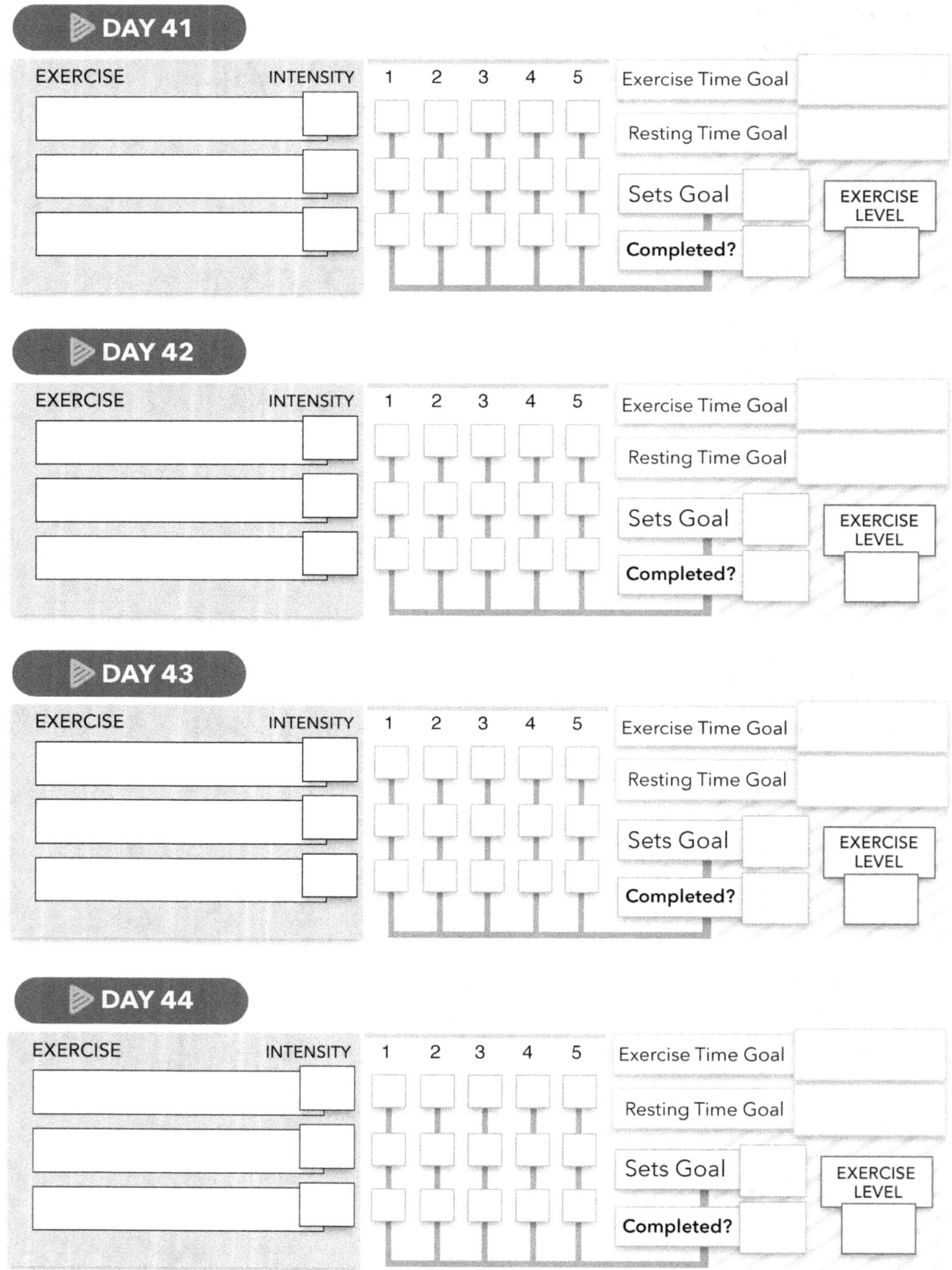

DAY 41

EXERCISE | INTENSITY | 1 2 3 4 5

Exercise Time Goal
Resting Time Goal
Sets Goal
Completed?
EXERCISE LEVEL

DAY 42

EXERCISE | INTENSITY | 1 2 3 4 5

Exercise Time Goal
Resting Time Goal
Sets Goal
Completed?
EXERCISE LEVEL

DAY 43

EXERCISE | INTENSITY | 1 2 3 4 5

Exercise Time Goal
Resting Time Goal
Sets Goal
Completed?
EXERCISE LEVEL

DAY 44

EXERCISE | INTENSITY | 1 2 3 4 5

Exercise Time Goal
Resting Time Goal
Sets Goal
Completed?
EXERCISE LEVEL

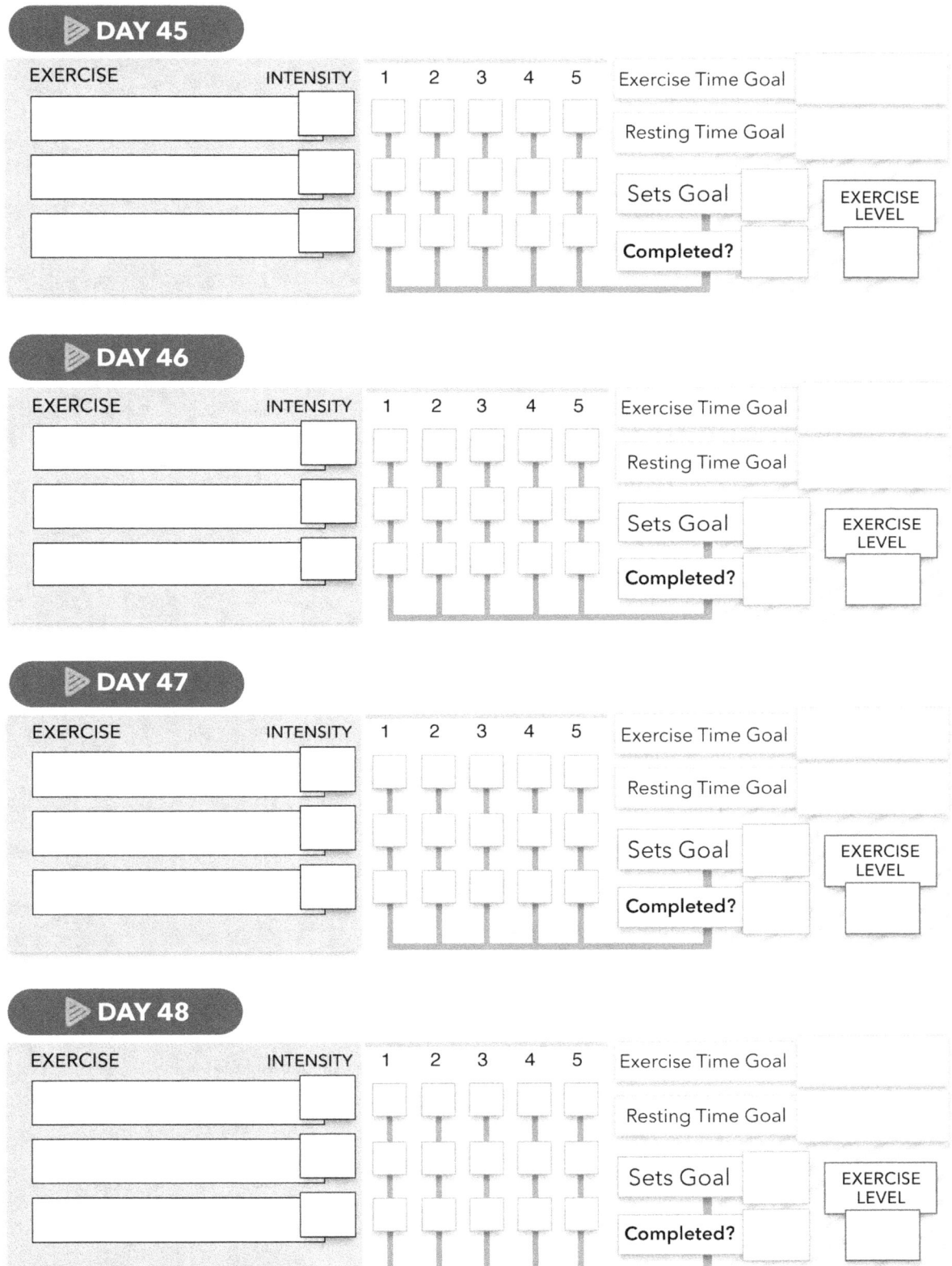

DAY 45

EXERCISE   INTENSITY

1   2   3   4   5

Exercise Time Goal

Resting Time Goal

Sets Goal

Completed?

EXERCISE LEVEL

DAY 46

EXERCISE   INTENSITY

1   2   3   4   5

Exercise Time Goal

Resting Time Goal

Sets Goal

Completed?

EXERCISE LEVEL

DAY 47

EXERCISE   INTENSITY

1   2   3   4   5

Exercise Time Goal

Resting Time Goal

Sets Goal

Completed?

EXERCISE LEVEL

DAY 48

EXERCISE   INTENSITY

1   2   3   4   5

Exercise Time Goal

Resting Time Goal

Sets Goal

Completed?

EXERCISE LEVEL

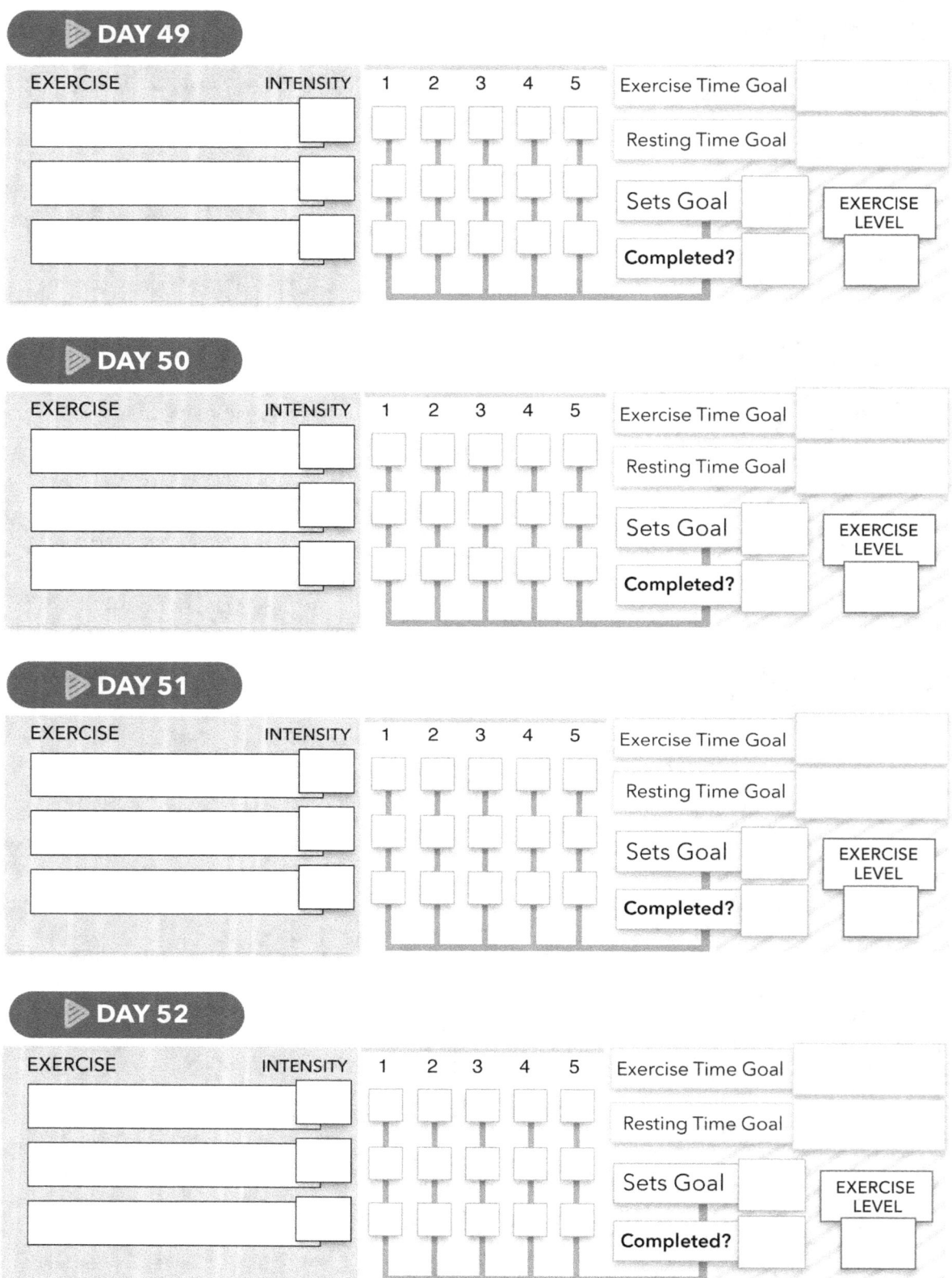

DAY 49

EXERCISE | INTENSITY

1 2 3 4 5

Exercise Time Goal

Resting Time Goal

Sets Goal

Completed?

EXERCISE LEVEL

DAY 50

EXERCISE | INTENSITY

1 2 3 4 5

Exercise Time Goal

Resting Time Goal

Sets Goal

Completed?

EXERCISE LEVEL

DAY 51

EXERCISE | INTENSITY

1 2 3 4 5

Exercise Time Goal

Resting Time Goal

Sets Goal

Completed?

EXERCISE LEVEL

DAY 52

EXERCISE | INTENSITY

1 2 3 4 5

Exercise Time Goal

Resting Time Goal

Sets Goal

Completed?

EXERCISE LEVEL

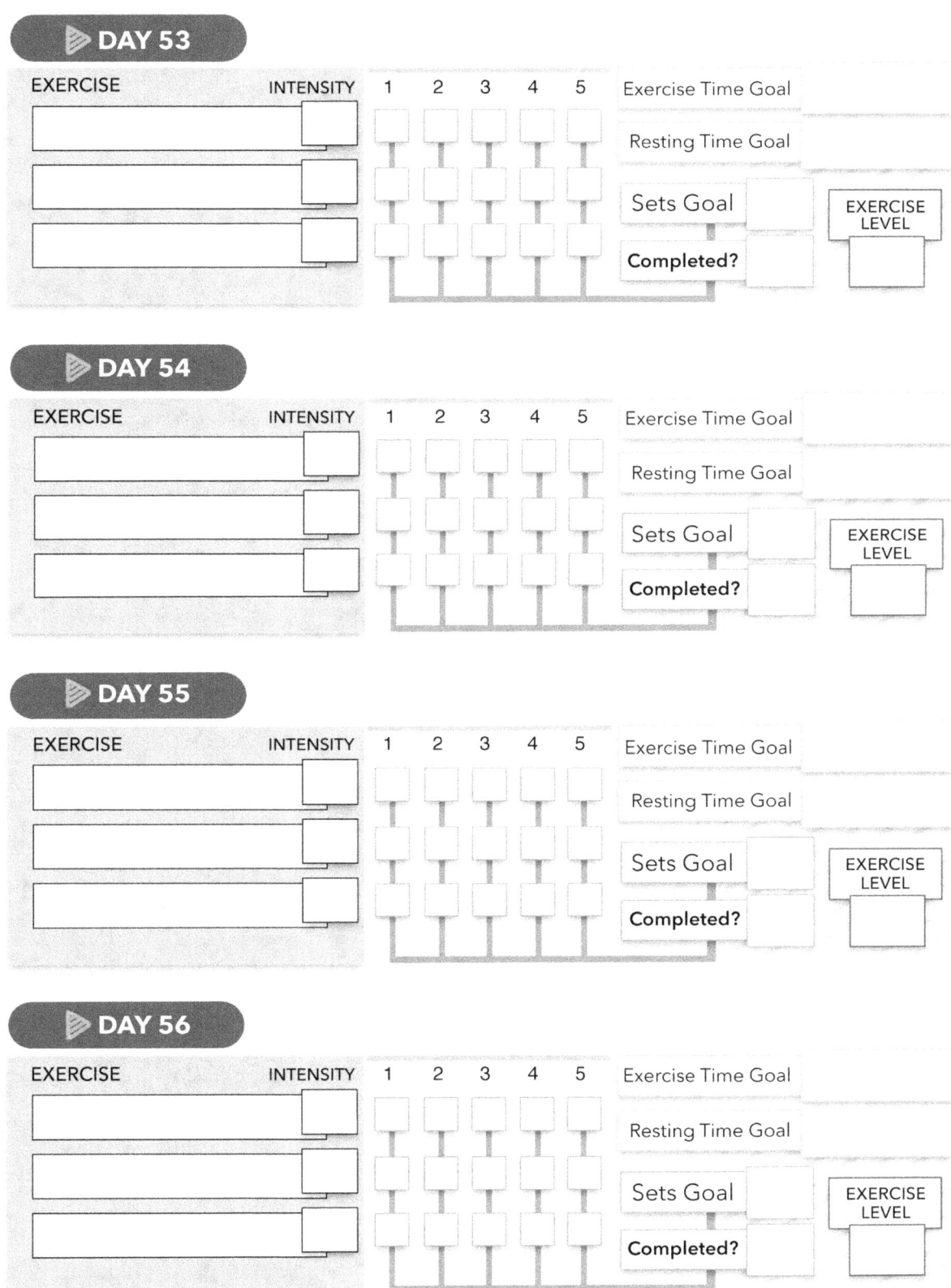

DAY 53

EXERCISE | INTENSITY | 1 2 3 4 5

Exercise Time Goal

Resting Time Goal

Sets Goal

Completed?

EXERCISE LEVEL

DAY 54

EXERCISE | INTENSITY | 1 2 3 4 5

Exercise Time Goal

Resting Time Goal

Sets Goal

Completed?

EXERCISE LEVEL

DAY 55

EXERCISE | INTENSITY | 1 2 3 4 5

Exercise Time Goal

Resting Time Goal

Sets Goal

Completed?

EXERCISE LEVEL

DAY 56

EXERCISE | INTENSITY | 1 2 3 4 5

Exercise Time Goal

Resting Time Goal

Sets Goal

Completed?

EXERCISE LEVEL

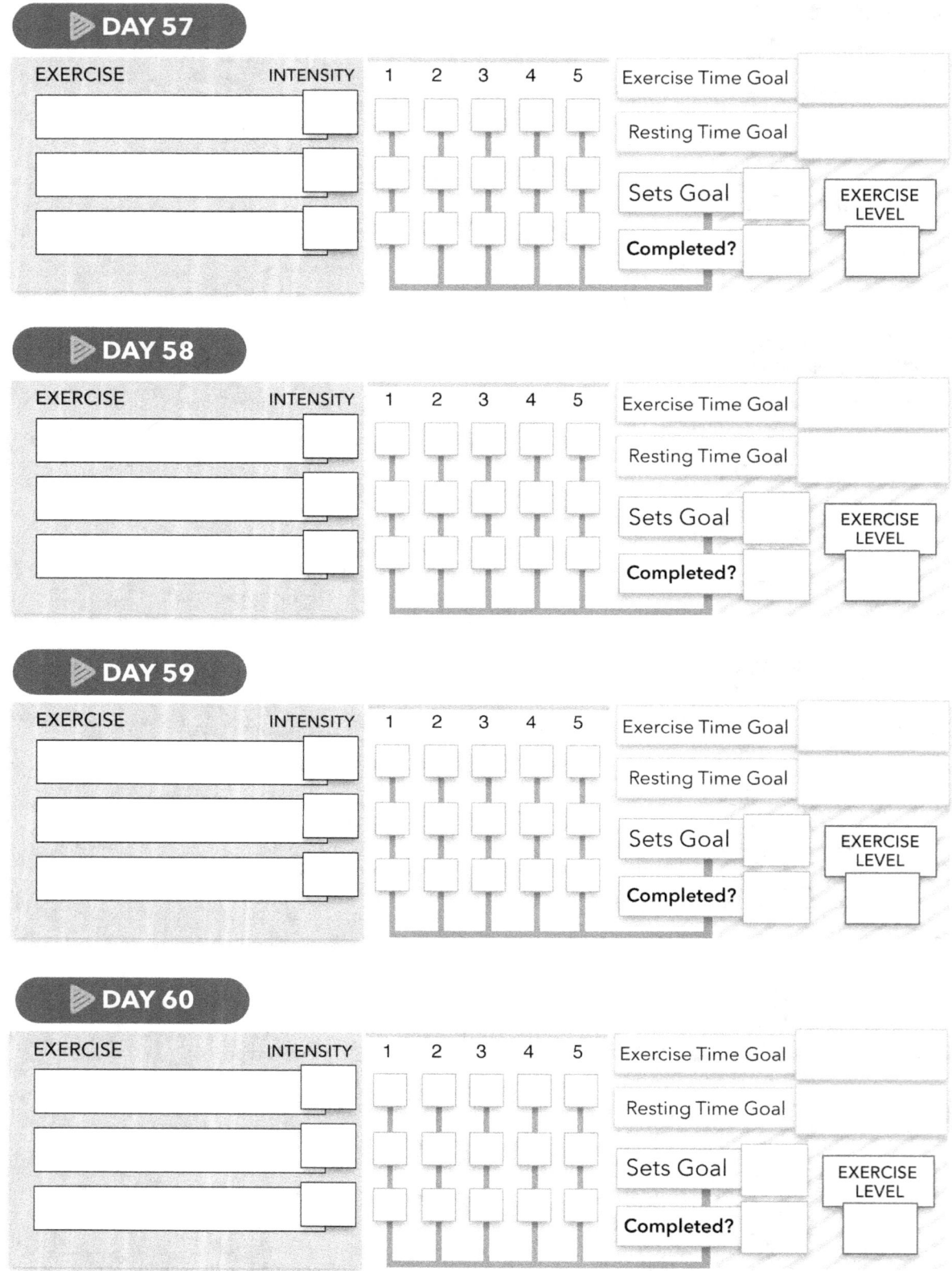

DAY 57

EXERCISE | INTENSITY

1 2 3 4 5

Exercise Time Goal

Resting Time Goal

Sets Goal

Completed?

EXERCISE LEVEL

DAY 58

EXERCISE | INTENSITY

1 2 3 4 5

Exercise Time Goal

Resting Time Goal

Sets Goal

Completed?

EXERCISE LEVEL

DAY 59

EXERCISE | INTENSITY

1 2 3 4 5

Exercise Time Goal

Resting Time Goal

Sets Goal

Completed?

EXERCISE LEVEL

DAY 60

EXERCISE | INTENSITY

1 2 3 4 5

Exercise Time Goal

Resting Time Goal

Sets Goal

Completed?

EXERCISE LEVEL

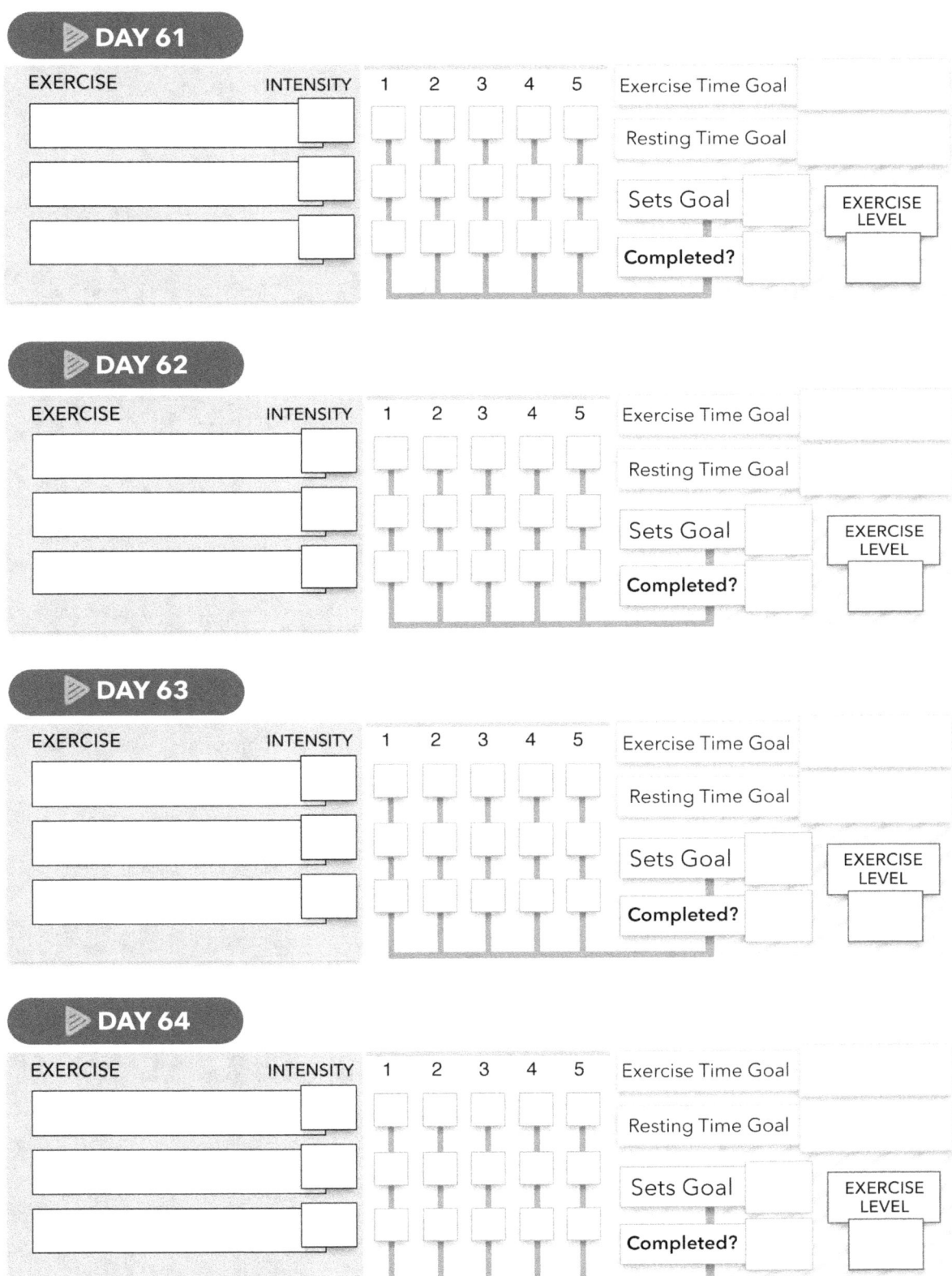

DAY 61

EXERCISE   INTENSITY

1   2   3   4   5

Exercise Time Goal

Resting Time Goal

Sets Goal

Completed?

EXERCISE LEVEL

DAY 62

EXERCISE   INTENSITY

1   2   3   4   5

Exercise Time Goal

Resting Time Goal

Sets Goal

Completed?

EXERCISE LEVEL

DAY 63

EXERCISE   INTENSITY

1   2   3   4   5

Exercise Time Goal

Resting Time Goal

Sets Goal

Completed?

EXERCISE LEVEL

DAY 64

EXERCISE   INTENSITY

1   2   3   4   5

Exercise Time Goal

Resting Time Goal

Sets Goal

Completed?

EXERCISE LEVEL

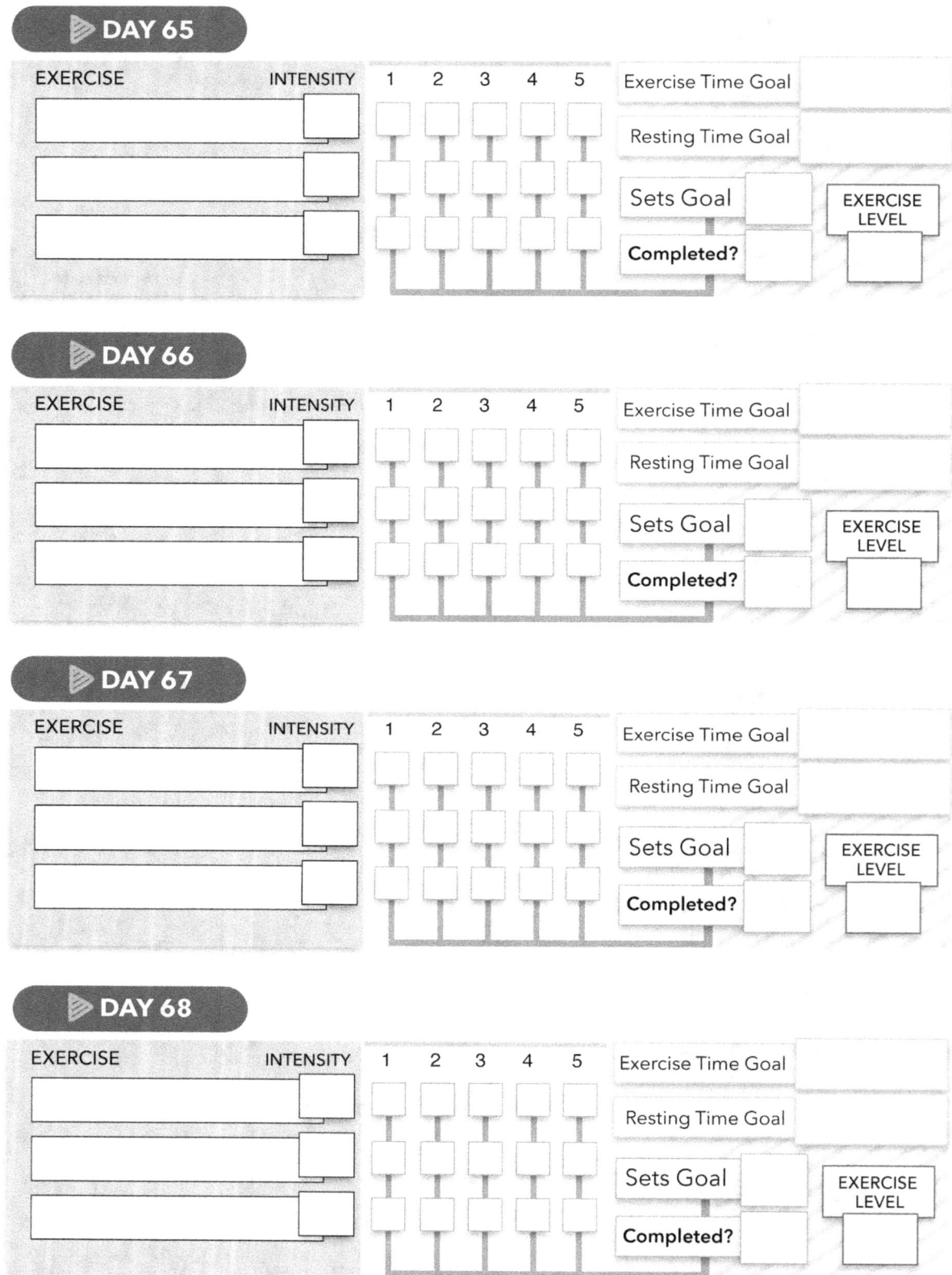

DAY 65

EXERCISE	INTENSITY	1	2	3	4	5

Exercise Time Goal

Resting Time Goal

Sets Goal

Completed?

EXERCISE LEVEL

DAY 66

EXERCISE	INTENSITY	1	2	3	4	5

Exercise Time Goal

Resting Time Goal

Sets Goal

Completed?

EXERCISE LEVEL

DAY 67

EXERCISE	INTENSITY	1	2	3	4	5

Exercise Time Goal

Resting Time Goal

Sets Goal

Completed?

EXERCISE LEVEL

DAY 68

EXERCISE	INTENSITY	1	2	3	4	5

Exercise Time Goal

Resting Time Goal

Sets Goal

Completed?

EXERCISE LEVEL

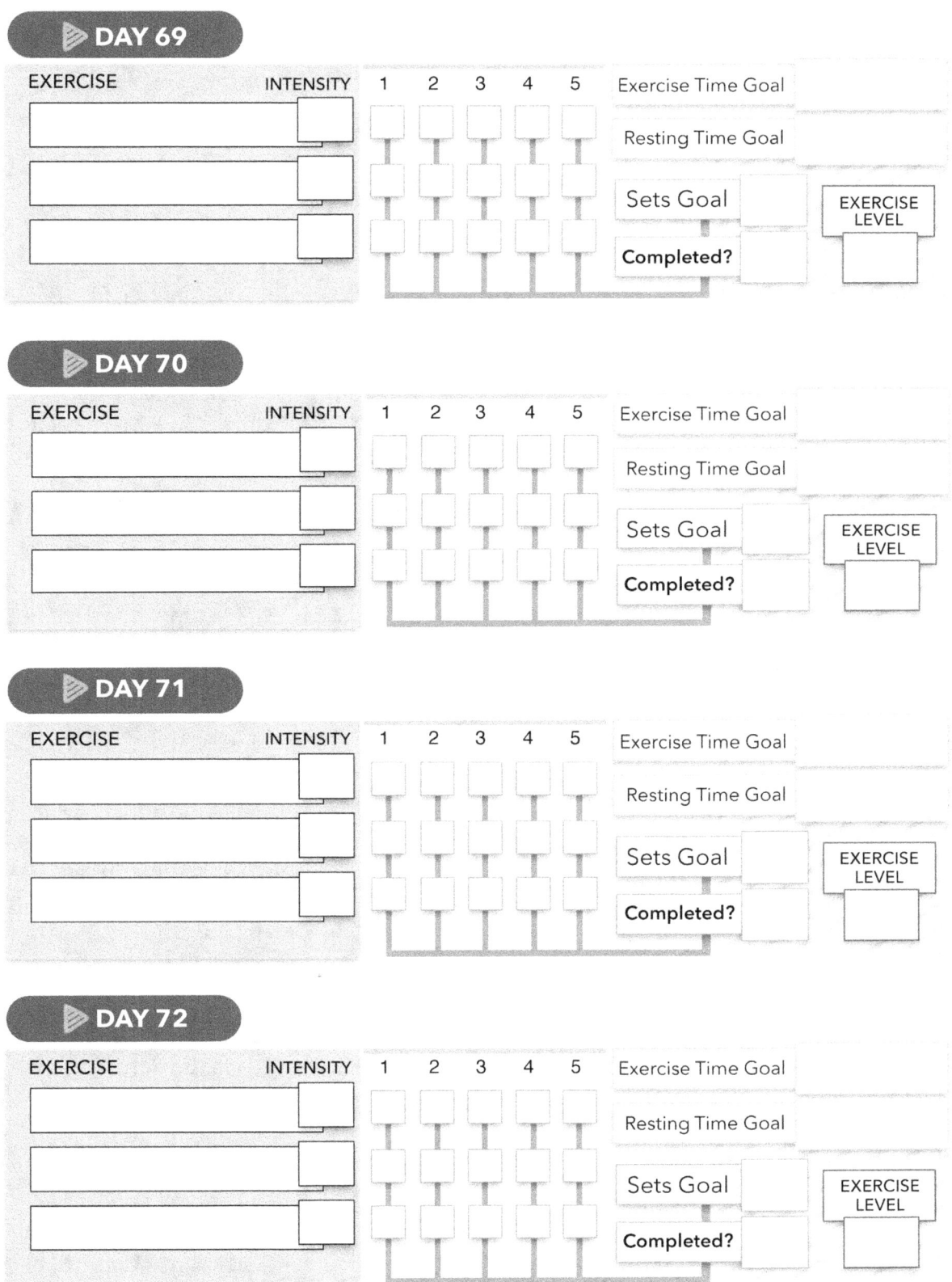

DAY 69

EXERCISE | INTENSITY
1 2 3 4 5
Exercise Time Goal
Resting Time Goal
Sets Goal
Completed?
EXERCISE LEVEL

DAY 70

EXERCISE | INTENSITY
1 2 3 4 5
Exercise Time Goal
Resting Time Goal
Sets Goal
Completed?
EXERCISE LEVEL

DAY 71

EXERCISE | INTENSITY
1 2 3 4 5
Exercise Time Goal
Resting Time Goal
Sets Goal
Completed?
EXERCISE LEVEL

DAY 72

EXERCISE | INTENSITY
1 2 3 4 5
Exercise Time Goal
Resting Time Goal
Sets Goal
Completed?
EXERCISE LEVEL

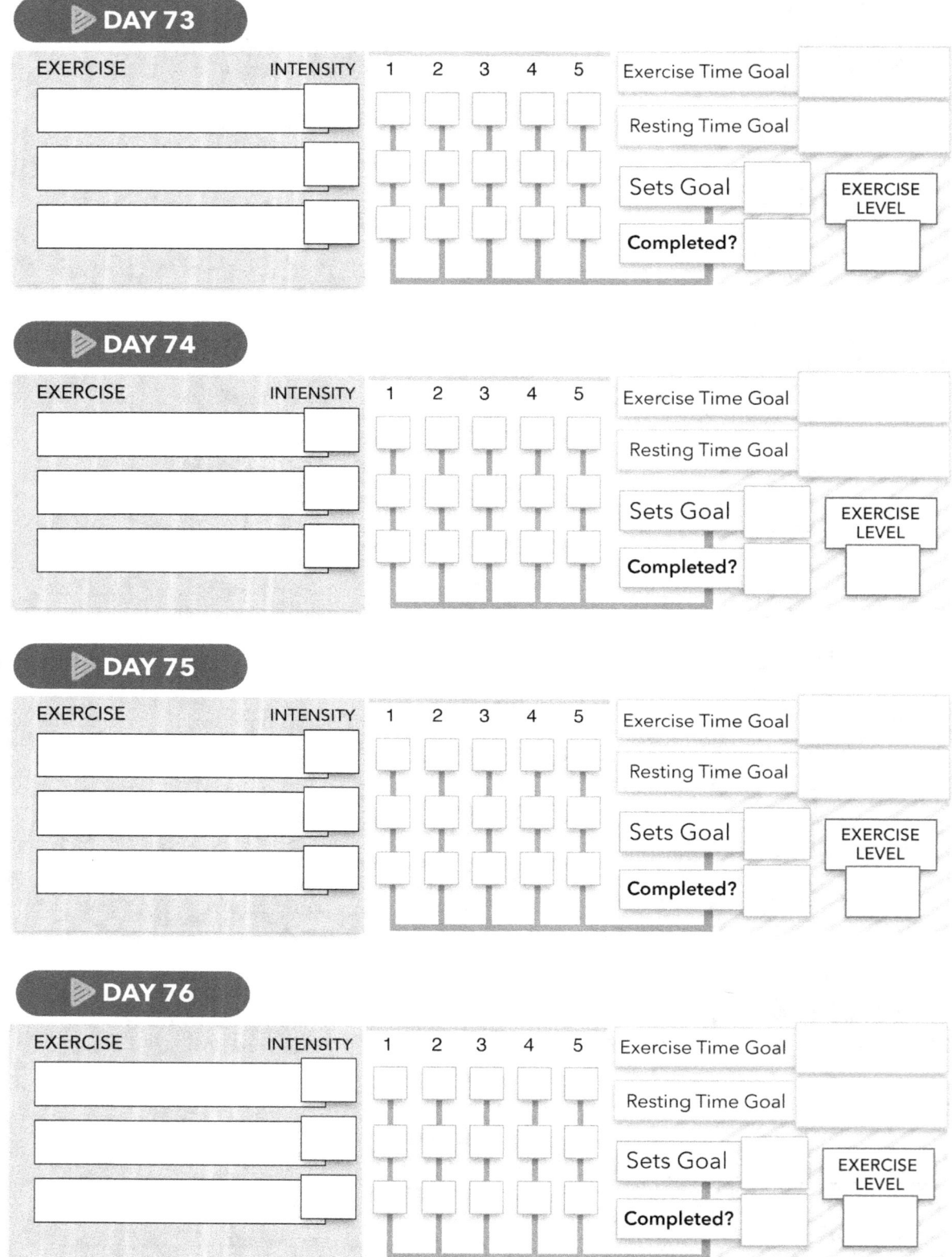

DAY 73

EXERCISE	INTENSITY

1	2	3	4	5

Exercise Time Goal

Resting Time Goal

Sets Goal

Completed?

EXERCISE LEVEL

DAY 74

EXERCISE	INTENSITY

1	2	3	4	5

Exercise Time Goal

Resting Time Goal

Sets Goal

Completed?

EXERCISE LEVEL

DAY 75

EXERCISE	INTENSITY

1	2	3	4	5

Exercise Time Goal

Resting Time Goal

Sets Goal

Completed?

EXERCISE LEVEL

DAY 76

EXERCISE	INTENSITY

1	2	3	4	5

Exercise Time Goal

Resting Time Goal

Sets Goal

Completed?

EXERCISE LEVEL

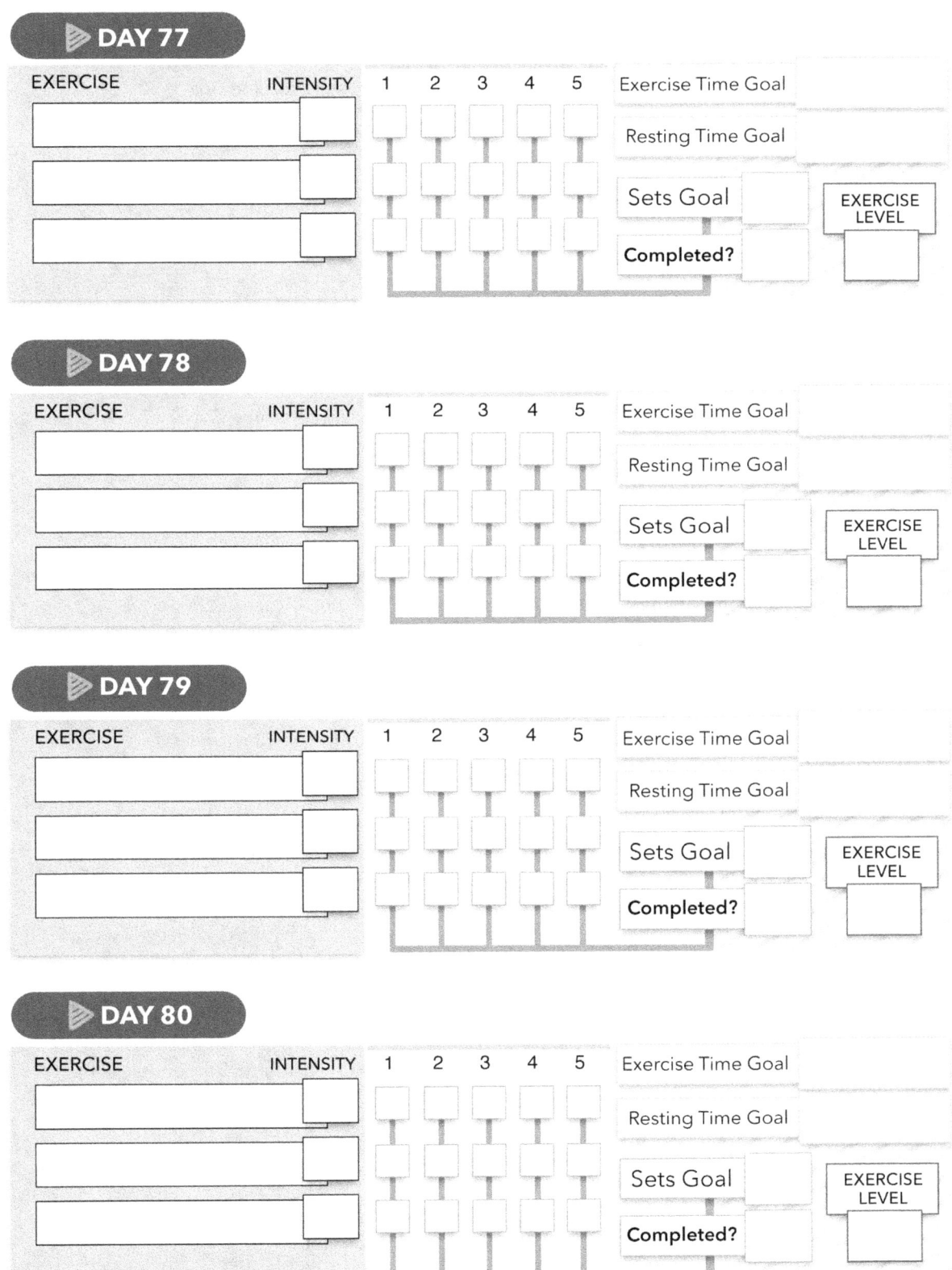

DAY 77

EXERCISE | INTENSITY

| | 1 | 2 | 3 | 4 | 5 |

Exercise Time Goal

Resting Time Goal

Sets Goal

Completed?

EXERCISE LEVEL

DAY 78

EXERCISE | INTENSITY

| | 1 | 2 | 3 | 4 | 5 |

Exercise Time Goal

Resting Time Goal

Sets Goal

Completed?

EXERCISE LEVEL

DAY 79

EXERCISE | INTENSITY

| | 1 | 2 | 3 | 4 | 5 |

Exercise Time Goal

Resting Time Goal

Sets Goal

Completed?

EXERCISE LEVEL

DAY 80

EXERCISE | INTENSITY

| | 1 | 2 | 3 | 4 | 5 |

Exercise Time Goal

Resting Time Goal

Sets Goal

Completed?

EXERCISE LEVEL

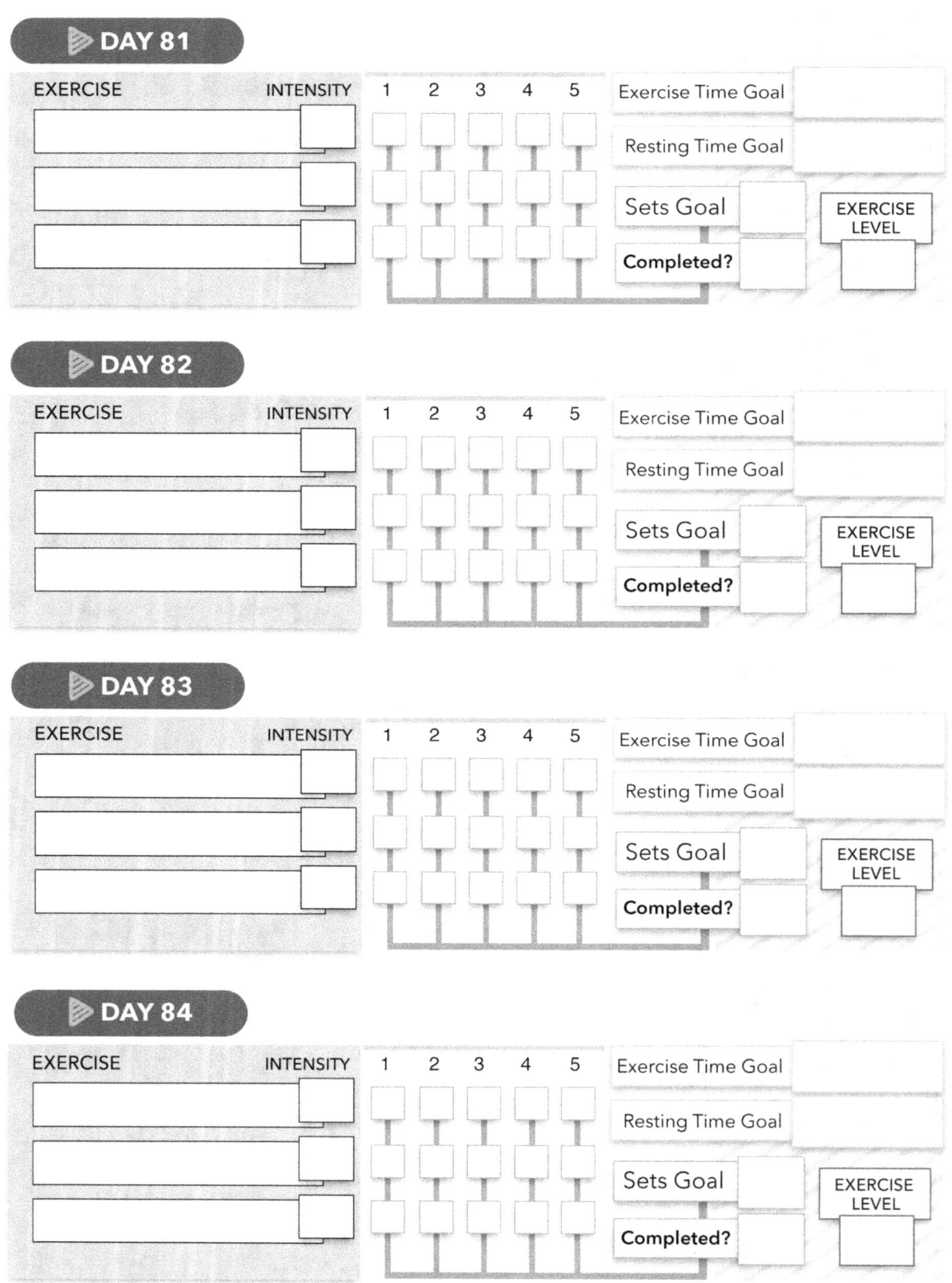

DAY 81

EXERCISE | INTENSITY | 1 | 2 | 3 | 4 | 5

Exercise Time Goal

Resting Time Goal

Sets Goal

Completed?

EXERCISE LEVEL

DAY 82

EXERCISE | INTENSITY | 1 | 2 | 3 | 4 | 5

Exercise Time Goal

Resting Time Goal

Sets Goal

Completed?

EXERCISE LEVEL

DAY 83

EXERCISE | INTENSITY | 1 | 2 | 3 | 4 | 5

Exercise Time Goal

Resting Time Goal

Sets Goal

Completed?

EXERCISE LEVEL

DAY 84

EXERCISE | INTENSITY | 1 | 2 | 3 | 4 | 5

Exercise Time Goal

Resting Time Goal

Sets Goal

Completed?

EXERCISE LEVEL

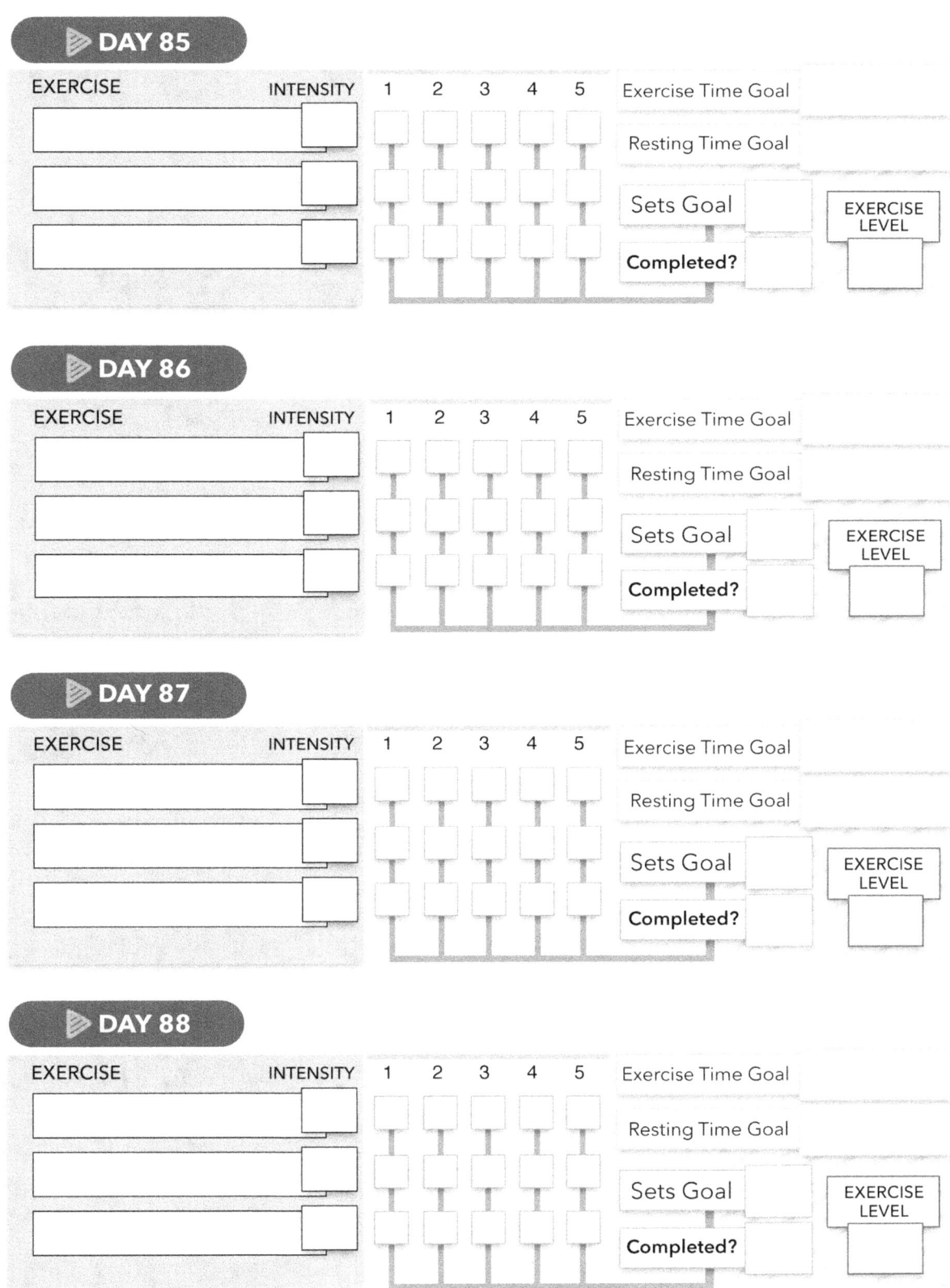

DAY 85

EXERCISE | INTENSITY

1 2 3 4 5

Exercise Time Goal

Resting Time Goal

Sets Goal

Completed?

EXERCISE LEVEL

DAY 86

EXERCISE | INTENSITY

1 2 3 4 5

Exercise Time Goal

Resting Time Goal

Sets Goal

Completed?

EXERCISE LEVEL

DAY 87

EXERCISE | INTENSITY

1 2 3 4 5

Exercise Time Goal

Resting Time Goal

Sets Goal

Completed?

EXERCISE LEVEL

DAY 88

EXERCISE | INTENSITY

1 2 3 4 5

Exercise Time Goal

Resting Time Goal

Sets Goal

Completed?

EXERCISE LEVEL

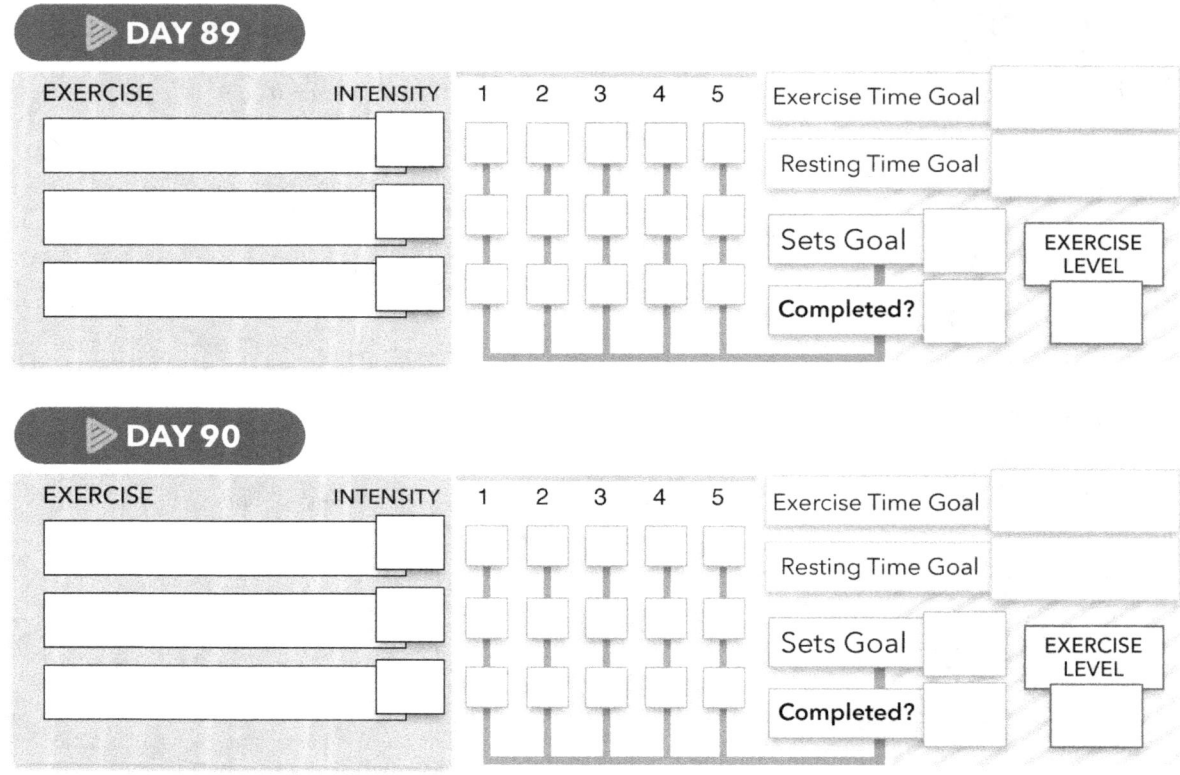

DAY 89

EXERCISE	INTENSITY	1	2	3	4	5

Exercise Time Goal

Resting Time Goal

Sets Goal

Completed?

EXERCISE LEVEL

DAY 90

EXERCISE	INTENSITY	1	2	3	4	5

Exercise Time Goal

Resting Time Goal

Sets Goal

Completed?

EXERCISE LEVEL

Another Day Complete

It matters not if you have a ✗ or ✔

You have completed another days routine.

Well Done You!

If it is Saturday – Enjoy tomorrow off!

EXERCISE PROGRESS CHART

	MONDAY	TUESDAY	WEDNESDAY	THURSDAY	FRIDAY	SATURDAY	SUNDAY
▷ WEEK 1							
▷ WEEK 2							
▷ WEEK 3							
▷ WEEK 4							
▷ WEEK 5							
▷ WEEK 6							
▷ WEEK 7							
▷ WEEK 8							
▷ WEEK 9							
▷ WEEK 10							
▷ WEEK 11							
▷ WEEK 12							
▷ WEEK 13							

☐ WE ARE ALL DIFFERENT

This is true, when it comes to weight loss and fitness, we all need something that is tailored to our body type and lifestyle. It's all too easy for someone to tell you how to run your life, what you should be doing and how you should be doing it. But they are not you. Only you are you, and you know what it feels like to be you!

I don't know you personally and I do not know your current weight and fitness goals. What I do know is, you are different from everyone else. You are you, special, unique and know your own abilities!

I know my own abilities and what I am capable off. I would like to think I could drive a formula one racing car! I mean how hard can it be? I drive all the time! But I know, deep down, I wouldn't make it around the first corner. Maybe after a little time, some professional coaching and determination I could make a lap of it?

☐ START AT THE BEGINNING

We all have to start at the beginning, regardless of the task! And when you are at the start you have to take it slowly, learn and grow! And before you know it, you become the master of your abilities.

Regardless of your goals, you have to find your own starting point and be honest with your own abilities. If you are, then your results will come quickly.

Remember, most of the time, the people who are the best at what they do are simply more organised with their approach. Now it is your turn to get organised and become the master of your own body. If you can organise your eating and exercise, you will be making an amazing change to your life. Whatever your goal, The Body Plan Plus 90 day plan will help you get there!

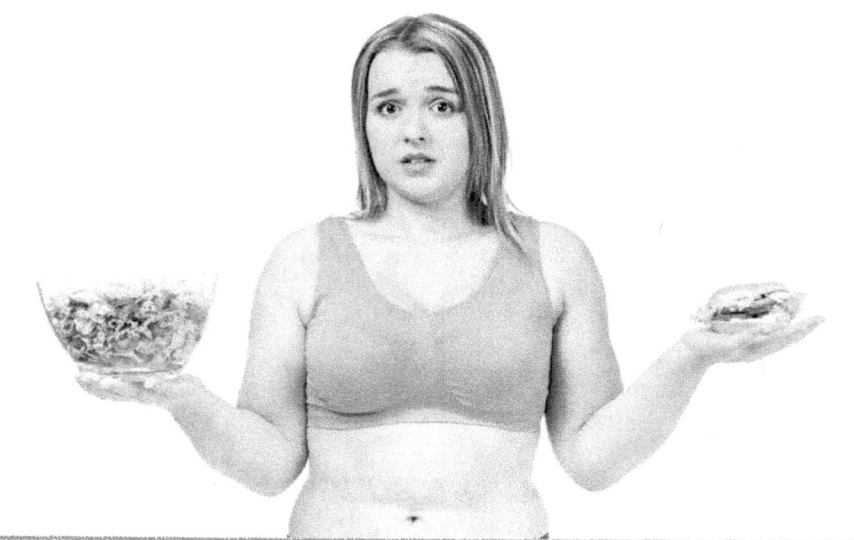

☐ BEING ORGANISED

We are all different and come in different shapes and sizes. Dependent on your activity levels, your fitness and stamina will differ greatly from someone who is of the same size and shape as you.

Your weight loss goal is also very different from others. Some people want to lose a few pounds or maybe a stone for a forthcoming Wedding or that summer holiday. And some people need to lose a lot more for their own health and well-being. Whatever the reason - A goal weight is on your mind!

There are many factors that make weight loss, fitness & stamina completely individual to us all. But this is often overlooked, and it feels like what is on offer to us in the weight loss and fitness world applies to the already fit and active. It's simply assumed that you are flexible, fit and able to perform high intensity exercises!

☐ GIVE UP POINTS

Just because an 11 stone person wishing to lose a few pounds can perform Burpee's and Jumping Jacks, does not mean a 17 stone person wishing to lose 5 stone can do the same. They may try, but after one workout session I'm sure they would not try again. Doing more than your ability will simply trigger "Give up points".

The same applies to dieting. If you are at the higher end of the weight scale, you burn more calories than someone at the lower end. So how can the same diet plan or club work for all, or be fair?
Answer: It can't!

Dieting, Weight loss and Exercise will not work for you, if you choose the wrong path. You have to make a plan that is right for you, and your body. You have to get organised for your calorie needs, your fitness levels, stamina and flexibility.

☐ WEIGHT LOSS IS FOR EVERYONE

*Weight loss and exercise is for everyone - Not just an already, thin, fit looking crowd! I think you know what I am talking about here! You've seen the commercials, Facebook and Youtube videos. Skinny athletic individuals jumping around without an ounce of body fat - **PROMOTING WEIGHT LOSS!***

It may work for you or a few individuals, but it will not work for everyone! Being honest and organised is the best place to start!

◆ YOUR THOUGHTS ON THE SUBJECT

☐ BEING HONEST WITH YOURSELF

The guide below is based on my own experiences, working out with various individuals of all shapes and sizes and various levels of fitness & flexibility. It has been proven to myself that we are all so different and in order to reach our own personal goals, we have to do something that is right for us as different individuals.

*When we think of exercise, we immediately picture a super fit aerobics instructor shouting out motivation, dancing around in front of us, with us trying to keep up with the pace! - Exhausting ! The key is to find something you can comfortably do, again and again, without triggering the **Give up points".***

If you are in the 10 to 12 stone weight range or less, everything in the weight loss and fitness world seems to fit around you. You can most likely perform any exercises out there, and all gym equipment works with your body structure. Dieting will also be a little easier for you, as you will not notice a reduction in Calories that much. The Body Plan Plus exercise programme would class you as a body type A person and will get you organised.

Interestingly, if you are in this weight range, you can be either or, fit or unfit! In this range you may be physically fitter than you think. You will have to pay close attention to how you feel the day after a workout. You may have to step up intensity or reduce it!
The Body Plan Plus exercise programme will help you get this right!

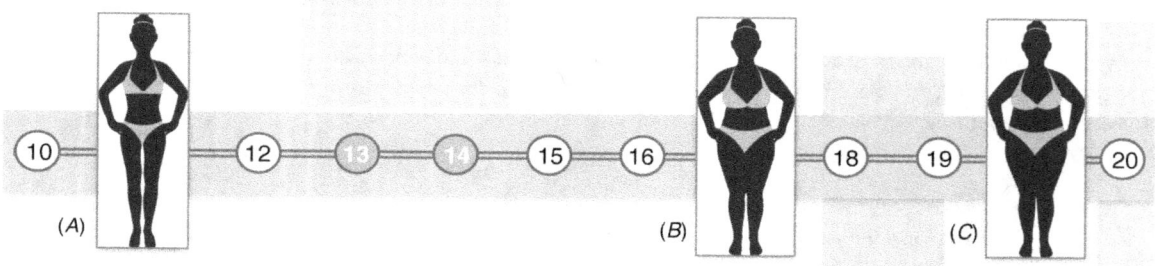

Beyond this weight range, other than swimming pools, the world of fitness seems to close the door to us. Help & guidance is limited - And it feels like you're on your own!

If you are currently in this range, you have to do things at a slower pace. Don't think for one minute you are not doing as much work as someone lighter than you. On the contrary, you will most likely be working harder and burning more calories. A little hard to explain in such a limited space, so watch the website video and I will explain why you will be working just as hard. The Body Plan Plus exercise programme will show you how to work out effectively without burning yourself out!

☐ FINDING YOUR GROOVE!

If you are at the lower end of the scale, you may think the rest of my "Waffle" does not apply to you?
Please read on because the fundamentals and formula for weight loss and fitness success applies to all.
All I am trying to do here is allow you to think about your body type, and what is right for you to begin with.

Regardless of your starting point, at the end of the day, your goal is to get to the lower end of the scale and get fit at the same time. If you are already close - it simply means you will get there a little quicker. That is, if you do the right stuff!

In the beginning it's a common mistake and all to easy to say - "Do more, push harder", but this "Much too soon" approach will simply trigger the "Give up points".

The fitness pros may cringe at what I am about to say, but sometimes "Plodding" along will get you the long term results you want. And I've seen this for myself. The slow "Plodder" comes back to the gym, again and again! And quite quickly they stop plodding, because their bodies need more and more! And so the cycle begins and miracles happen!

If you do something your body isn't used to, it's going to let you know about it. You will become fatigued very quickly, and the prospect of performing the same exercise routine the following day will be far from your mind.

☐ SMALL EFFORTS

If it's easy and makes us feel good, then we do it again and again.
And it's this continuing pattern of "Small Efforts" many times over that will get us the results you want.

☐ The key to long term fitness and weight loss - is long term!

You have to build exercise and fitness into your life everyday, and to achieve this, you have to find the right balance for your body. Remember: You are going to be reducing your calories as well as exercising, so we have to take it slowly.

▷ *Don't be prey to the industry pros, pushing you to do more than you should be, otherwise you will simply fall victim to the - too much effort vs. little reward!*

◆ YOUR THOUGHTS ON THE SUBJECT

☐ EFFORT VS. REWARD

It seems like nowadays, anyone promoting weight loss and fitness exercises are simply showing off!

The harder and more complex the exercise mechanics are, the more it seems to pushed as a "Must do exercise".

If you have no point of reference to exercising, you would think - "How can I possibly do that"?

> *This frustrates me greatly because the promoters of such exercises, do not take into account your age, flexibility, body shape, current stamina or fitness level. If you haven't been over active for some time, your tendons, ligaments and muscles (Including your heart) could be a little out of tune. So if you jump in at the deep end and attempt to perform silly exercises, there is a chance you could do yourself some damage.*

The truth is, you don't need to kill yourself by jumping around like a "Wild monkey" to burn calories. That is, not until your body is ready for it.

As you progress with your exercises, and your stamina increases beyond the slower gentle exercise range - then yes, get prepared to hit it hard!

To start with, gentle repetition over "Too Much Effort" works every time. It's more productive to perform gentle calorie burning exercises everyday, than bursts of high intensity that leave you feeling exhausted.

High intensity and flexible challenging exercises do burn more calories per minute, but there's not much in it. And if your body isn't used to them, you will ache and be in pain - this will trigger the "Give up" points you so desperately want to avoid.

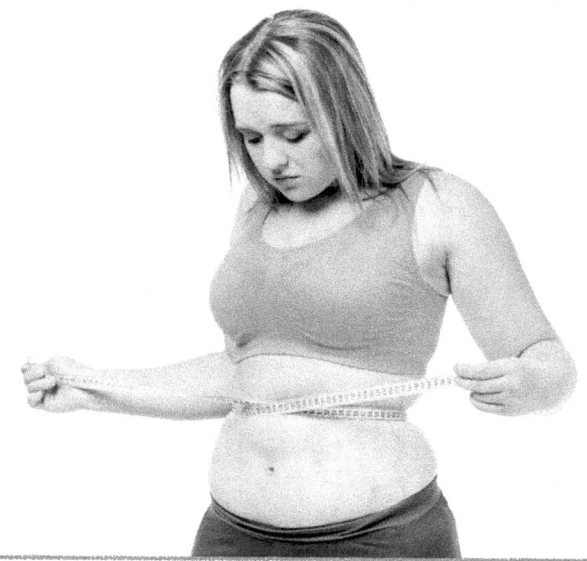

☐ HONEST EATING

How many times have you decided to change the way you eat?

You tell yourself "This is it, I have the latest healthy recipe book, and I'm sticking to it". A week and half later that new book finds a home for itself on the kitchen window sill next to last year's dusty top sellers!

So what goes wrong? Nine times out of ten it is just the fact that all the recipes in these new books feature ingredients you just don't have or are not used to buying. I recently looked at one book which had recipes for squid and scallops: Where do you keep your squid? This is not what I call "Honest" everyday eating.
Honest eating is exactly that!

Don't get me wrong, there are some books out there that do focus on wholesome everyday food that your Mum and Gran used to make - and hats off to these chefs!

> ▷ *This isn't a cook or recipe book and I am not going to tell you what you should be eating. You should already know what's a healthy option and what isn't. And I'm sure you already know fruit and vegetables are good for you!*

Trying to maintain something that's new is a little difficult, especially when it comes to food. You have to factor in your budget, your kids, time and effort. Sometimes the cheapest and easiest option seems to be the winner!

You want to lose weight, but you don't want to feel like you are on some kind of "Crazy diet". So you have to think smart and focus on weight loss in a different way.

Calorie control is the key answer. And that means you can eat exactly what you like providing you don't go over your daily calorie allowance. It will not take you long to work out some foods contain less calories, allowing you to eat more of them and still stay within your daily calorie allowance.

In time when you lose more weight and get fitter, you will naturally start to select the healthier more filling foods. Foods that give you energy, boost your metabolism and all round make you feel better.

But just like everything else, don't rush in and jump from what your used to, to something "Exotic and fruity".

Take it slow, give it some thought and get it right!

◆ YOUR THOUGHTS ON THE SUBJECT

THE SHOPPING LIST

Because you are about to watch and monitor you calorie intake, you will start to research the many more food options that are out there. You will read about good and bad calories, high fibre, low and high carbs and super foods. But remember, don't get drawn into buying stuff you don't need just yet.

To ensure your success, you have to live comfortably with your shopping trolley. Its contents can sometimes be the make or break of your diet. Just because you're on a diet, it does not mean your trolly has to be over flowing with fruit and vegetables. It would be great if it did, and in time it will begin to look rather healthy. But one step at a time!

It would be nice to say - Everyone should start the day with a great nutritional breakfast with fruit sprinkled over your oats. But making the world's most exotic breakfast is far from your mind when you are rushing around in the morning and for practical reasons your cornflakes come top of the list.

> When you're tracking your calories this does not matter. As long as your cornflakes are measured out and weigh the correct amount according to your "Calorie Library", your diet is going to be a success.

It would be nice to have the healthier option everyday, but if you're honest you just can't. Try and get it in as many times as you can, but don't worry and feel like you have failed if you don't!

Over time you can start to make various changes to your foods. You can look at your list and say to yourself "What's a better option, but not much of a change" ?

On your shopping list pages you will find "boxes to tick" for low, medium and high Calorie items. Use your judgment and make changes when you're ready. Swap high Calorie items for lower healthier versions. And that can be as follows:

Big brand Cornflakes to Healthier Cornflakes.
Healthier Cornflakes to Oats - Oats to better Oats.
Better Oats with fruit and so on... Get the idea?

Honest eating is going to make you feel like you're not on a diet - All you have to do is just remember to count the calorie value, write it down and stick to your Daily Calorie Goal.

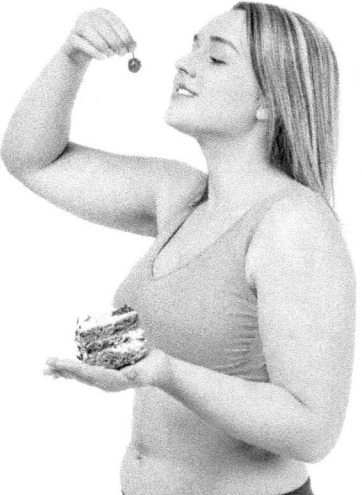

☐ YOUR CALORIE GOAL

The figure you put in this box is very important! (In fact the most important part of your weight loss programme.) If you put the figure too high, you may not lose weight, but gain it and if you put the figure too low, you will lose weight, but it will be uncomfortable.

The key to successful and long term weight loss is to lose weight at a rate that is not noticeable to you mentally or physically. In other words, not feeling starved or deprived. Diets fail because if you are not getting enough calories you will feel fatigued and miserable - and then simply give up!

*It is said, a healthy balanced diet for an "**Average**" man to maintain his weight is 2,500 calories and for the "**Average**" woman it's 2000 calories. "These values will vary depending on age, metabolism and levels of activity".*

*To lose a healthy pound of body weight each week, these "**Average**" people would have to reduce their daily calorie intake by 500 calories. So, for "**Average**" men it will be 2000 calories and for average women it's 1500.*

*The highlighted and important word here is - "**Average**"!*

*Chances are if you are looking to lose some weight, you may not be average, so we need to find out the amount of calories **YOU** need to lose weight. And at the same time feel good about it and not deprived.*

Many people will not research this enough to know how many calories their body needs, so they simply go for the "Average" - and come up with 1500 calories - big mistake!

*Everyone is different and we all come in different shapes and sizes, tall, short, big & small boned and of course big & small, or "fat or skinny". Regardless of your body type we need to calculate how many calories **YOU** need to feel content and lose weight.*

For some of you it may be the average 1500 calories, and for others in may be a lot more! The great advantage calorie control has over dieting/food plans is calorie counting allows you have to more calories if you need them.
And together we can work this out!

Some of us need more calories than others! And if you are at the higher end of the weight scale, you most likely need more. And this is not because you are greedy, but simply a larger body needs more energy to fuel itself.
A larger body can mean "More fat mass" or "More muscle mass" or a combination of both.

Your body needs fuel constantly. We don't have to be on the move all the time to burn calories, we burn them all day long for just being alive, and this is called your BMR "Basal Metabolic Rate".

◆ YOUR THOUGHTS ON THE SUBJECT ⎯⎯⎯⎯⎯⎯⎯⎯⎯⎯⎯⎯⎯⎯⎯⎯⎯

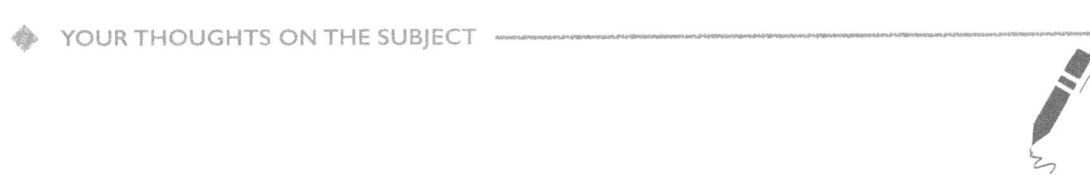

☐ YOU CAN'T SIMPLY SAY

So you can't simply say to yourself "My calorie goal is 1500" (The average) otherwise you may be reducing your calorie intake by too much and you will struggle.

*If you have a higher **BMR**, you need to adjust your calorie intake accordingly. If you don't, you may feel deprived and reach for that chocolate treat. In doing so, you will feel guilty and think - "I have failed".*

*But you would have only failed with your calorie goal calculation, because you would have believed you went over it, when in fact you had plenty left, because your **BMR** is higher than the average!*

*It can be confusing because there are so many factors to consider when calculating the correct amount of calories you need as an individual. You body is different from somebody else's, and if you get it wrong, you will feel hungry all the time. We want to avoid this major "**Give up**" trigger point.*

☐ MUSCLE BURNS A LOT OF CALORIES

The amount of calories we burn at rest is mostly dependent on our muscular size. Muscles use up a lot of energy, and the more muscle you have the more energy you burn. Regardless of any eating habits, you have been getting protein in your diet. We all know Protein builds muscle!

So if you have some spare body fat, chances are you have an extra few pounds/kilos of muscle mass too! That extra muscle will be in the form of extra thigh & calf muscle.

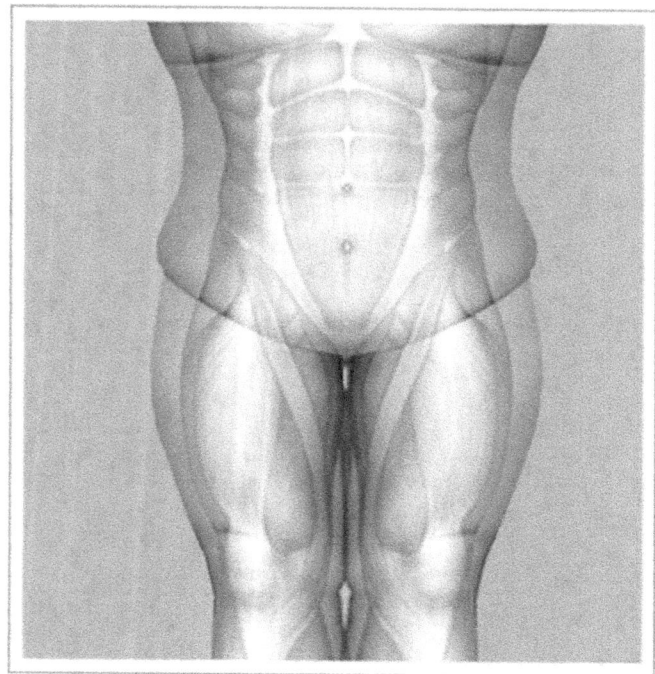

SPARE BODY FAT

So if you have some spare body fat, chances are you have an extra few pounds/kilos of muscle mass too!
That extra muscle will be in the form of extra thigh & calf muscle.

SAY HELLO TO HELEN & SOPHIE

This can be clearly demonstrated with these two very different individuals, Helen and Sophie, after using a body composition analyser.

▷ *Helen's Fat Mass is **47.1kg**, while Sophie's is **24.6kg**   (**22.5kg** Difference)*

▷ *Helen's muscle mass is **61.3kg** and Sophie's muscle mass is **44.1kg** (**19.2kg** Difference)*

▷ *Helen has a **BMR** of **2039** Calories, while Sophie's is only **1400** Calories (**639** Calorie Difference)*

*If we added the activity calories to each individual, lets say **600 Calories each**, and then subtract their **500 Calorie deficit** for weight loss, the results we look like this:*

Helen

Weight 18 Stone 5lb (117.7kg)
Weight Loss Goal 4 Stone
Fat 42.2%
Fat Mass 47.1kg
Muscle Mass 61.3kg
Bone Mass 3.3kg

BMR	*2039*
Activity Calories	*600*
Daily Maintenance	*2639*
Calorie Deficit for weight loss	*500*
Daily Calorie Goal	**2139**

Sophie

Weight 11 Stone 2lb (71.1kg)
Weight Loss Goal 1 Stone
Fat 34.6%
Fat Mass 24.6kg
Muscle Mass 44.1kg
Bone Mass 2.4kg

BMR	*1400*
Activity Calories	*600*
Daily Maintenance	*2000*
Calorie Deficit for weight loss	*500*
Daily Calorie Goal	**1500**

◆ YOUR THOUGHTS ON THE SUBJECT

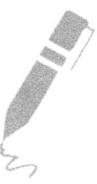

Being at the lower end of the weight scale, Sophie is pretty much "Average" and Helen is not.

If both put in 1500 calories as a starting point, Sophie would think, "What's all the hassle about? Dieting is easy".   Helen would find it harder, because her Calorie reduction would be over 1100 Calories!   This clearly is not fair and why many diets and food plans fail. A dieting club would argue, Helen could eat as many "Vegetables" as she wanted to make up the short fall.   But even a bucket of broccoli weighing 3 kilos still isn't going to match it! (Not to mention being very unpleasant).

SO... HOW DO YOU GET YOUR BMR?

There are various on line BMR calculators, but the one we recommend is linked to our website: www.thebodyplanplus.com (Clients Area) "BMR Calculator".

All you have to do is enter some basic information, Gender, Age and Weight.

You will also be asked your activity level, be honest as this will affect your results.
Saying you are more active than you are will result in more calories being added to your total.

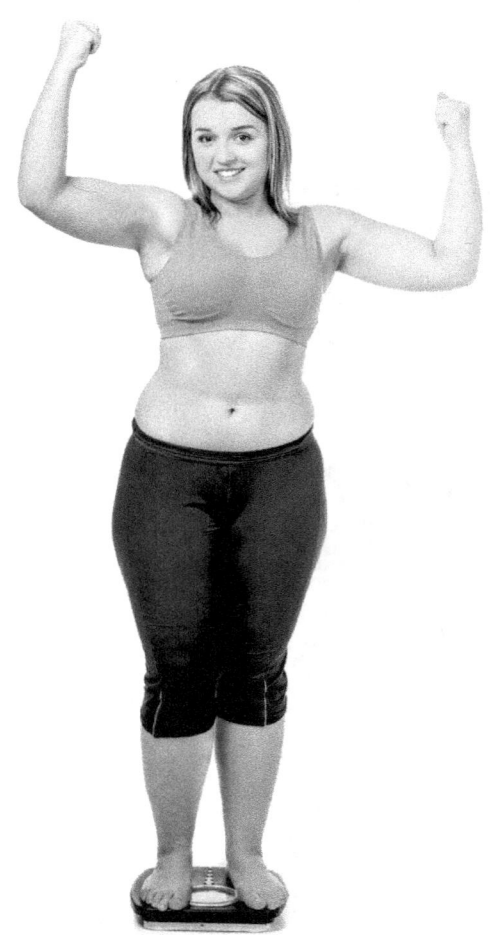

*You will be given two figures: Your **BMR** and your Daily Calories allowance,*

Take the second figure, your daily Calorie allowance and deduct 500 Calories.

*The figure you get will be your **NEW CALORIE GOAL**.*

As discussed on the previous page. The calculation hasn't factored in your Muscle mass, so it may be out a little. But don't worry too much about this, because at the end of the day it's a better place to start than just choosing the 1500 average. If our calculations are out by too much.... Don't worry there is a fix for this!

*If you want a truly accurate **BMR**, use a Body Composition Analyser. See page 185 for more information or visit our website.*

☐ HOW MUCH?

If we have got your **BMR** figure right and the calculations correct, you should lose a healthy pound of body weight each week.

If we have got the calculations wrong, and factor in heavier muscle mass, don't worry! All you have to do is juggle with your daily calorie goal. If you are losing too much weight, simply add some calories to your daily calorie goal and if you are not losing weight, then reduce the figure.

If you have to do this, do it sparingly and adjust the figures by 150 Calories either way.

If you listen to your body, then you are going to get it right. Remember, your weight loss hasn't got a time scale to it. You want to make the changes without noticing it! Very much like with the weight going on, you want to it come off at a rate that's not noticeable.

This does sound rather boring, maybe not as fast as you would like, but trust me, it is faster than you think!

☐ IT WENT ON, SO IT CAN COME OFF!

The extra body weight you have gained, whether 1 stone or 4, didn't get here overnight. It was a slow process and you didn't notice it. The body you have now, will feel like it's the body you have always had. And this is simply time **OVER** small amounts, on a regular daily or bi-daily basis.

If you know your body, look back on photos taken a few years ago, you will see the increase. Maybe, you have weighed yourself over time and know how much you weighed last year, or the year before? If you do, then you can calculate how many Calories "Over" you have been consuming on a daily basis.

You will be surprised that it is not really that many.

They say a pound of body fat is 3500. It is a guideline and there is debate over the actual figure. But for practical reasons and without boring you with thermo-dynamics, we will stick with 3500 Calories.

If anyone has been gaining weight at a rate of half a pound every two weeks, then that's a yearly weight gain of 13 pounds (1 pound short of a stone).

This means that this person would have only been consuming roughly 900 Calories per week more than they should. If these Calories were consumed proportionally throughout the week, it only works out to be around 130 Calories per day. **WOW!** That's not a lot at all!

> **BUT IT IS**, when you consider this. Standing in the line waiting for your regular "Coffee" you're tempted by the snack size flap jack without knowing it contains 250 calories…. And you haven't got your 140 Calorie coffee yet!

> If you are not conscious about your calorie intake, it really is easy to go over! Hopefully, with the knowledge you have just gained, and using your Body Plan Plus Diary, this will not happen to you. You will be in control!

☐ WHY DO WE NEED TO EXERCISE

Exercising makes us fit and healthy. It's what we do, to simulate what our ancestors did a long time ago. Some people don't have to exercise at all because their day to day activities are just so energy demanding, they can eat as much and as often as they like and look pretty fit, trim and healthy. These individuals have found their body balance. The energy (Calories) they consume is equal to the energy (Calories) they burn.

These individuals are usually heavy labourers and are constantly using their muscles. For the rest of us to get to the same level of energy output, we have to play sports or hit the gym and exercise!

Sometimes it's forgotten what exercising is all about! It is often thought of as a sport people do simply for fun and to look good. But if you really think about it, it is an essential way of life. If your day to day living is not burning off the energy (Calories) you consume, then it's something you have to do to keep your body balanced. And if you don't, well you know what happens!

There are a number of reasons why we don't all have gym memberships; "It's not my thing", "I can't afford it", "I'm not fit enough", "I don't have time", "I don't want to look silly", "I can't perform those exercises". The list is long!

> ▷ *Thousands of people sign up to a new Gym Membership every January. They go almost four to five time a week for about 3 weeks, then this reduces to once a week for a week or two. And then they don't return!* **Why?**

Working out at home can sometimes offer up even more reasons not to be doing it. Sometimes the intention is there and the motivation simply isn't. That's why many of us have dusty exercise bikes in the corner of the room, doubling up as a clothes horse!

You need motivation and a solid reason to exercise five days per week and because you don't have a personal trainer knocking on your door at 7.30am, it's all up to you! Now you have the reason, you simply need the motivation.

But you can do it! And with The Body Plan Plus Exercise Programme, it will be easier than anything you have tried in the past. The ease of it and the results will be the motivation you are looking for!

You will feel like you can perform your new routine every day in double quick time and this is good news. This programme will fit around your lifestyle, no matter how busy you are!

☐ JUST LIKE MAGIC!

Diets and Exercising do not fail, they work! What fails us is our starting point. If you do something your body isn't used to, it will simply tire. You get all the signals rushing to your brain telling us, "This is to much" - "I don't like it" and "Don't do it again".

You get these signals, (Feelings) because you try to do something your body isn't ready for yet. To prepare your body for anything, you have to do it at a pace that allows it to adapt! You have to do something that is easy, and not too taxing for you, emotionally as well as physically.

> *A little scenario for you to prove my point! If you had a magic red button and to lose a pound of body fat each week, all you had to do is push it repeatedly for **20 Minutes** last thing at night. Would you push it? Of course you would, and you would not miss a single day until your goal weight was reached! And why would you never miss a day? Because it's so easy and effortless!*

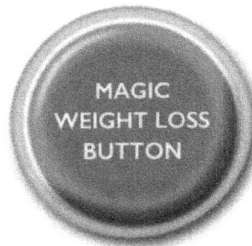

*So! We have now proven, if it's easy, you will do it again and again until your goals are reached. We have also learnt you are prepared to dedicate **20 Minutes** of your time for the task.*

But how can we make exercising easy? "It's hard isn't it? I've seen people jumping around like they are on fire" and that looks difficult! These individuals are not on fire, they have simply reached a level where, what they are doing is still quite easy to them, and they feel good about it. But they too had a starting point!

It's all about the starting point and what your body is capable of doing! You need to do something slowly and at a pace your body will thank you for. And if you do, you will get the right signals rushing to your brain "This is easy", "This is fun", "I feel good", "I want to do it again" "I feel motivated"!

The exercise formula you are about to read about will show you an easy starting point for your body type and how to increase or reduce your intensity.

This will allow your body time to adapt to the small changes, and pushing your body to next level when its ready to…. Thus making it as easy as pushing a magic button.

☐ CREATE YOUR OWN EXERCISES

Exercise is about movement and making your muscles work a little harder than normal. Muscles respond and burn energy from repetition (Continuous movement) and or tension from lifting weight (Force against gravity) Your body is weight, so therefore various movements force your body to act against gravity.

For example: Getting up from a sitting position causes your thigh muscles to contract as you put your upper body weight on them! Your thigh muscles have to contract for just a moment, but if you repeat the process continuously they will call upon more energy to keep the movement going - The heavier you are, the greater the force against gravity and the harder your thigh muscles will have to work, and thus burn more energy.

A lighter person could perform more repetitions than a heaver person. So once again, not all exercises are equal, and it looks like the larger person just isn't putting in the effort - But believe me they are, if not more!

If you are heavier or have limited flexibility, you can take an existing exercise movement, and reduce its range of motion to make it easier and fair.

> ▷ *Remember, it's all relative and the effort required matches your body weight and structure, so the Calorie burning is equal to the amount of energy you require to work against gravity.*

I have created two new exercises that do this. People with lower flexibly or heavier bodies will be able perform these moves more comfortably and burn just as many calories, if not more! Half Jacks (An easier version of jumping jacks) and Quarter Squats (An easier version of squatting) See Body Plan exercises pages.

Feel free to create and invent your own exercises. All you have to do is ensure your muscles are under tension, and tire if you repeat the movement many times. If you invent an exercise that you can do pretty fast, without losing balance - then that's even better! Let me know the mechanics of your new exercise and we will put them up on our website for others to try.

Remember, exercise is not about working out to complete exhaustion! Getting fit, increasing your stamina and all round health will come faster with repetition. Exercising lightly, every day or as many days possible will be more beneficial than a burst of "Over doing it".

Pushing yourself beyond your limits is a common mistake and will simply produce - **Negative Results**
No matter how fit you are!

SUMMARY - WHERE DO YOU GO FROM HERE?

Weight loss and fitness is a continuous endeavour. In the beginning it can seem like a real challenge and your will power may be tested on many occasions. It is a bit like everything in life and when you are the beginning it's hard and maybe a little scary! Over time you become the master of it and it becomes easy and fun. It really does!

It's a wonderful "Catch 22", the fitter and thinner you become the more you want to push yourself. The more you push yourself the healthier you get! It really will happen for you to! Remember, small honest steps first. Know your body and what it's capable of. Listen to your body and don't change too much to soon, because if you do you could potentially fail.

In time you will find your body balance, and you will be eating what your body needs to fuel itself. Sometimes you will need less and sometimes more. You will no longer notice food, and you will be focused on quality and not quantity. You will become conscious about what you are eating and you will want to fuel your body with healthier options and this will make you feel good.

You will want to do more exercise and take the longer routes. Calorie burning tasks from house work to gardening will no longer seem a challenge. In fact you will not notice walking mile after mile and everything becomes easy to achieve.

*Keep it up, keep tracking your foods and recording your exercise progress. Think of yourself as a growing tree - throughout the difficulties that lay in your path, you will flourish and **you are beautiful.***

Additional information - Body Composition Analyser

Getting your BMR using "Body Composition Analyser" is highly recommend. The results you get will be stop on. You also get a good look to see what your made of! The information is super valuable and includes, the amount of fat around your organs, body fat percentage and total fat weight, muscle mass percentage and total muscle weight, the weight of your bones and more….

It's easy to do! Simply slip off your shoes, stand on the scales and hold two side bars for 30 seconds. Some health food stores such as Holland and Barrett offer this service for a few pounds. They print out the results for you and believe me the information is well worth the money.

Calorie Library Calculations - Calories Per Single Gram

To make life easy, the calorie value should be a single unit. Then it's simply to calculate the calorie value. Example: If your Ham slices are 1.2 Calories per gram, and they weight 49.8 grams, then the calculation would be 49.8 x 1.2 = 59.76 Calories.

Round it up to make life easy and your Ham Slices have the calorie content of 60 calories.

How to break down your calorie value to a single unit. If something is 49 calories per 100 grams, simply divide the value (49 calories) by 100 grams and you get the answer. (49 divided by 100 = 0.49 calories)

If the item weights 163 grams, you now know the formula, 163 x 0.49 = 79.87 Calories. Round it up for an easy life! And it's 80 Calories!